Interpreting
Radiographs

Interpreting Trauma Radiographs

Jonathan McConnell
Head of Medical Imaging
Christchurch Polytechnic Institute of Technology
New Zealand
formerly
Principal Lecturer
Medical Imaging Sciences
St Martin's College
Lancaster and Carlisle, UK

Renata Eyres
Associate Dean for Academic Enterprise
Faculty of Health and Social Care
University of Salford, UK

Julie Nightingale
Director of Postgraduate Studies
Senior Lecturer (Radiography)
Faculty of Health and Social Care
University of Salford, UK

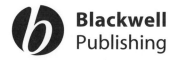

Blackwell
Publishing

Editorial offices:
Blackwell Publishing Ltd, 9600 Garsington Road, Oxford OX4 2DQ, UK
  Tel: +44 (0)1865 776868
Blackwell Publishing Inc., 350 Main Street, Malden, MA 02148-5020, USA
  Tel: +1 781 388 8250
Blackwell Publishing Asia Pty Ltd, 550 Swanston Street, Carlton, Victoria 3053, Australia
  Tel: +61 (0)3 8359 1011

First published 2005 Blackwell Publishing Ltd

Library of Congress Cataloging-in-Publication Data
McConnell, Jonathan.
    Interpreting trauma radiographs / Jonathan McConnell, Renata Eyres, Julie Nightingale.
        p.   ;   cm.
    Includes bibliographical references and index.
    ISBN-13: 978-1-4051-1534-6 (pbk. : alk. paper)
    ISBN-10: 1-4051-1534-3 (pbk. : alk. paper)
  1. Wounds and injuries – Diagnosis.   2. Wounds and injuries – Imaging.
3. Diagnosis, Radioscopic.
    [DNLM: 1. Wounds and Injuries – radiography.   2. Bone and Bones – injuries.   3. Bone and Bones – radiography.   4. Pattern Recognition, Visual.
5. Radiography – methods.] I. Eyres, Renata.   II. Nightingale, Julie.   III. Title.

    RD93.7.M38 2005
    617.1'07572 – dc22

                                                          2005000283

ISBN 10: 1-4051-1534-3
ISBN 13: 978-14051-1534-6

A catalogue record for this title is available from the British Library

Set in 10 on 12 pt Sabon
by SNP Best-set Typesetter Ltd., Hong Kong
Printed and bound in Great Britain
at CPI Bath Press, Bath

The publisher's policy is to use permanent paper from mills that operate a sustainable forestry policy, and which has been manufactured from pulp processed using acid-free and elementary chlorine-free practices. Furthermore, the publisher ensures that the text paper and cover board used have met acceptable environmental accreditation standards.

For further information on Blackwell Publishing, visit our website:
www.blackwellpublishing.com

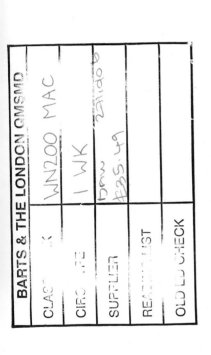

Contents

Preface

The editors of this book have acquired several years experience in the curriculum development and management of masters' level programmes, focused particularly to developing and enhancing image reporting skills in non-medically qualified health care practitioners. Although we originally designed such programmes to serve the needs of reporting radiographers, our education provision has evolved to encompass other health professionals who wish to develop reporting skills, including emergency nurse practitioners, physiotherapists and podiatrists.

Through the work outlined above we identified a need for a key text which could be recommended to support the education and training of radiographers and other health professionals in acquiring the skills of image reporting. Although a number of excellent associated texts are available, it was felt that they are either prohibitively expensive, too complex or too simplified, or do not address the full spectrum of the reporting practitioner's needs.

In designing *Interpreting Trauma Radiographs* we have attempted to present the reader with a firm underpinning knowledge of the scientific basis of plain radiograph skeletal reporting, including pattern recognition, decision-making, anatomy and physiology, as well as the pathomechanics of trauma. We have also attempted to document the historical journey which has shaped the UK radiography reporting service into it's present form, such that we have a better understanding of the potential inter-professional conflicts and resistance which may still be encountered today, particularly outside the United Kingdom.

However, we firmly believe that such conflicts are easily overcome by ensuring a rigorous approach to the education, clinical training and assessment of reporting practitioners. As outlined in our legal aspects and radiologist's perspectives chapters, safe delegation of reporting requires practitioners to be well-educated, assessed as competent to practice both within the clinical department and educational setting, supported by their employer from a medico-legal standpoint, and offering evidence of continuing competence in reporting.

To support the development of practical report-writing skills we have offered chapters subdivided into the different regions of the skeleton. These chapters have been written with the novice reporting-practitioner in mind, leading the reader through the key concepts of each anatomical area, mechanisms of injury, resulting trauma patterns and related paediatric concerns. However, we also hope that *Interpreting Trauma Radiographs* will be of value to experienced practitioners, who may wish to use the text as a reference source in view of the extensive pathology index.

We have attempted to extensively illustrate the key concepts with radiographs, line drawings, tables and flow-charts, and we would like to encourage the student to revise and recap on their knowledge by reviewing the enclosed radiographs, attempting to describe the full image appearances, and then accessing additional information in the self-test answer boxes. These have been placed upside-down to avoid the tendency for cheating!

We hope that *Interpreting Trauma Radiographs* will be of use not only to reporting radiographers and those training for this role, but also to casualty medical officers and doctors in training, accident and emergency nurse practitioners, and other health professionals involved in the care of trauma patients.

We would like to express our sincere gratitude to the following organisations and individuals, without whom this book would not have been possible. Our thanks go to Blackwell Publishing and in particular to Caroline Connelly (Commissioning Editor), Sophia Joyce and Sally Rawlings for guiding us patiently through the publishing process. Our thanks also to the University of Salford (Greater Manchester) and the University College of St. Martins (Lancaster), for the loan of their extensive radiographic image libraries. Finally, our most grateful thanks go to Amanda Martin of the University of Salford and Bolton Royal Hospitals Trust, for proof reading and validating the work. Amanda is the seemingly tireless and enthusiastic course leader for a range of reporting programmes at the University, as well as being a reporting radiographer with many years experience in both adult and paediatric trauma settings. Her balanced and knowledgeable contributions have enhanced the work considerably, and we are most grateful for her input.

We have thoroughly enjoyed compiling *Interpreting Trauma Radiographs* and hope that you, the reader, find it a useful text to support your reporting activities.

Julie Nightingale
May 2005

1 Introduction

Jonathan McConnell and Julie Nightingale

In the past decades the reporting of medical images in the UK has remained firmly in the domain of radiologists, with radiographers legally prevented from expressing an opinion on radiographs by the 1922 Society of Radiographers Articles of Association. However, an important climate change occurred around the mid-1990s, mainly in response to the well-documented acute shortage of radiologists[1] leading to criticism of aspects of the reporting service provided by departments[2]. This was reflected in a number of publications by professional bodies that outlined clearly the benefits of redefining and developing the radiographer's role[3,4] and hastened the introduction of guidelines which were later to facilitate such developments. In particular, the College of Radiographers document entitled *Reporting by Radiographers: A Vision Paper*[3] was seen as pivotal to the success of radiographer reporting. In this document the professional body clearly supported the advancement of the radiographer's scope of practice, stating that 'Reporting by radiographers is not an option for the future, it is a requirement'. In 1995, a highly critical Audit Commission report noted the failure of radiology departments to provide a report on all examinations, many being received too late to influence patient management. Indeed, in the Ionising Radiations (Medical Exposure) Regulations (2000), there is now a requirement to ensure that there is a clinical (radiological) evaluation following each medical exposure.

According to the Special Interest Group for Medical Image Interpretation (SIGMII) protocols[5], the examinations most likely to remain unreported (or reported too late) are plain film examinations. In this field, particularly in trauma and orthopaedics, it was recognised that radiographers had already begun to develop considerable preliminary skills in abnormality detection, in part due to the adoption of the 'red dot' system of abnormality flagging by many departments. A number of academic institutions in the UK consequently developed postgraduate plain film reporting courses that concentrated on skeletal trauma and orthopaedics[6]. Such courses are now well established throughout the UK, and trauma reporting has firmly moved into the domain of radiographers. In many hospitals radiographers now undertake a high proportion of the plain film reporting workload, with an increasing emphasis on immediate or 'hot reporting' in Accident and Emergency settings.

In many other countries across Europe, North America and Australasia, development of radiographer and technologist reporting skills is also gaining momentum. In the UK the practice of radiographer reporting is no longer limited to radiologists and radiographers. Increasingly nurse practitioners, casualty officers, physiotherapists and other health professionals are also actively engaging in formalised reporting, guided by appropriate protocols.

We (the editors of this textbook) have several years' accumulated experience in the development and delivery of our respective institution's postgraduate reporting courses. The spectra of these programmes include trauma and orthopaedics, chest and abdominal radiography, gastrointestinal reporting, mammography image interpretation and progression towards cross-sectional image interpretation. We have also been actively involved in national reporting related activities, including validation and approval of postgraduate programmes, external examiner duties at other institutions, and involvement on the committee of the multidisciplinary SIGMII (formerly Special Interest Group in Radiographic Reporting). Such activities have highlighted the need for a key text to support the education and continuing professional development of practitioners from all disciplines who are involved in the reporting of skeletal radiographs. A range of useful texts is currently available, but we have found that the cost of some of these texts is prohibitive and we believe that others are over-simplified for postgraduate purposes or advanced training.

This textbook has therefore been compiled to incorporate information to assist the radiographer or practitioner engaged in reporting of trauma radiographs of both the appendicular and axial skeleton (as we do not believe that they can be studied in isolation). Although we have not specifically concentrated upon pathology other than trauma, we have made reference to those pathologies encountered in general radiographic practice.

The book is divided into two sections. Section One (Chapters 2–6) begins with some important general and background reading, providing an essential knowledge base on which to build reporting practice. In Chapter 2, Professor Nigel Thomas considers the historical background of radiographer/practitioner reporting from a radiologist's perspective, and he discusses the main elements of a radiographic report. Nigel has been an advocate of radiographer reporting for many years and a leading force in the development of reporting programmes and the establishment of SIGMII. In Chapter 3 Professor Bridget Dimond considers the legal framework within which radiographers and other practitioners will report. Bridget, a barrister with a special interest in legal aspects of health and social care, highlights in particular issues concerning accountability and negligence. Dr Ian Christensen, a psychologist with a keen interest in the psychological aspects of perception and interpretation, then explores the science underpinning how we view a radiograph and the decision-making pathways that we create (Chapters 4 and 5). In the final chapter in this section (Chapter 6), Julie Nightingale explores the fundamentals of musculo-skeletal anatomy and physiology required for the interpretation of plain films. She discusses the general clinically focused issues related to all areas of the skeleton, including mechanisms of injury, bone and joint trauma, and related pathologies.

The second section (Chapters 7–12) focuses on image interpretation of specific anatomical areas. It has been presented in such a way as to support reporting practitioners in training as well as providing a useful resource for those more experienced in reporting practice. The chapters, authored by Renata Eyres and Jonathan McConnell, lead the reader through the range of frequently encountered injury patterns, outlining the common pitfalls that may face the reporting practitioner. Specific anatomical and pathological patterns of injury are discussed and illustrated extensively with radiographic images and supporting diagrams, tables and charts. The radiographic images of trauma and pathology are accompanied by inverted captions (self-test answers), which will enable the reader to conduct self-tests while reviewing specific chapters. Chapters 7 and 8 present a thorough overview of a range of injuries afflicting the upper and lower limbs, perhaps the 'bread and butter' of radiographic reporting practice. Chapters 9 and 10 outline the range of trauma and pathology commonly affecting the spinal column and pelvis, an area increasingly incorporated into the domain of practitioner reporting on skeletal radiographs. Chapter 11 provides the practitioner with an overview of the complexities of the chest and bony thorax, specifically in relation to the diagnosis and interpretation of chest trauma. The last chapter (Chapter 12) discusses the role of plain films in the evaluation of trauma to the skull, facial bones and mandible.

Finally, we have included an index of trauma and pathological conditions to enable the practitioner to effectively use the text as a 'quick reference' tool for clinical practice, and as such we hope that it will be a companion guide during reporting sessions. We also hope that the lists of references and further reading in the chapters will also help to inform and support the practitioner in the development of the reporting role, enabling them to better fulfil the expectations of an advanced or consultant practitioner role in the future.

We hope that the text will be a valuable source of information for the following professional groups.

- Radiographers experienced in skeletal reporting and those training for this role.
- Student radiographers and qualified radiographers undertaking professional development activities, including those undertaking 'red dot' reporting.
- Medical practitioners, in particular casualty officers and orthopaedic doctors.
- Emergency nurse practitioners, particularly those engaged in referral for radiographic examinations.
- Physiotherapists and other professional groups, such as podiatrists, who have an interest in musculo-skeletal trauma and pathology.

One

We have enjoyed compiling this textbook, and we hope that readers will find it of great benefit to themselves and their colleagues. We welcome discussion and comments about any of the issues raised within this text. Our electronic contact details, and those of relevant organisations, are listed below.

Email addresses and websites

Jonathan McConnell: mcconnellj@cpit.ac.nz
Renata Eyres: R.D.Eyres@salford.ac.uk
Julie Nightingale: J.Nightingale@salford.ac.uk

The Society and College of Radiographers website: www.sor.org/
Special Interest Group in Medical Image Interpretation, Chair Dr D
   Manning: D.Manning@ucsm.ac.uk
Trauma Imaging Group, Chair B Snaith: tig_uk_chair@hotmail.com

References

1   Royal College of Radiologists (1995) *Statement on Reporting in Departments of Clinical Radiology.* RCR, London.
2   Audit Commission (1995) *Improving Your Image. How to Manage Radiology Services More Effectively.* HMSO, London.
3   College of Radiographers (1997) *Reporting by Radiographers: A Vision Paper.* CoR, London.
4   Royal College of Radiologists and College of Radiographers (1998) *Inter-Professional Roles and Responsibilities in a Radiology Service.* RCR/CoR, London.
5   Paterson, A.M., Price, R.C., Thomas, A. and Nuttall, L. (2004) Reporting by Radiographers: a policy and practice guide. *Radiography*, London, **10**(3), 205–11.
6   Prime, N.J., Paterson, A.M. and Henderson, P.I. (1999) The development of a curriculum – a case study of six centres providing courses in radiographic reporting. *Radiography*, London, 5(2), 63–70.

Further reading

College of Radiographers (1998) *X-ray Examination Requests by Nurse Practitioners and Radiographic Reporting by Radiographers.* CoR, London.
Price, R.C. (2001) Radiographer reporting: origins, demise and revival of plain film reporting. *Radiography*, London, 7(2), 105–17.

Section One

2

A Radiologist's Perspective

Professor Nigel Thomas

Through briefly outlining the historical context this chapter will consider the concept of other health professionals undertaking image reporting from the radiologist's perspective. It also outlines how to approach image interpretation and the process of formulating a report.

'Radiographers reporting? Over my dead body'

The above, unattributable quote was heard in the corridors of 38, Portland Place, London (the home of the Royal College of Radiologists) in early 1999. While the strength of the view is unmistakeable, it is far from original. The role of non-medical staff reporting on X-ray films has, in fact, been a subject of intense debate since Roentgen's discovery was made widely known in early 1896.

Immediately after the discovery of X-rays, their application to the practice of medicine became a 'tug-of-war' between the many interested parties. Relatively soon, however, there developed a distinct dividing line between those who produced the films (a diverse group including physicists, hospital porters, army orderlies, photographers, pharmacists and doctors), and those who felt able to offer an interpretation of the 'shadowgrams' which were produced. The medical profession initially wished to control both facets of the process, but it soon became clear to them that the most intellectually rigorous (and financially rewarding) part of the process was that of applying the interpretation of the images to patient management. This prompted the following anonymous statement in the *British Medical Journal* in 1903:

> There is no reason for professional prejudices against the practice of radiology by lay-men, so long as they confine themselves to the mere mechanical act of producing a picture and abstain from assuming scientific knowledge of the bearing of their radiographs on diagnosis or prognosis.

7

Two

Furthermore, the medical protagonists of radiology were keen to promote their new field as a genuine speciality in its own right. The recognition of radiology by the main stream of medical practitioners was, however, a slow process, prompting Thurstan Holland to state in 1917:

> There is a prevalent idea abroad that a radiologist is a mere photographer, and that any medical man can interpret radiographs. Never was there a greater mistake. The techniques of plate taking can be easily acquired by anyone; the more experienced one has become in the interpretation of radiographic findings the more conservative one becomes, and the more guarded in expressing dogmatic opinions.

The widespread use of X-rays during the First World War meant that there was a large number of non-medically qualified army personnel who had the ability to produce radiographic images. The end of the war threatened to flood the country with these individuals wishing to apply this knowledge in order to make a living. When discussing these military X-ray assistants, the British Medical Association was prompted to state that:

> A good many of them have acquired more self-confidence in diagnosis than is good for them or for the general public . . . the practice of medical radiography by lay persons, except under the direct instruction of medical practitioners, ought not to be encouraged.

As always, some people want to go that little bit further and, in a statement echoing the thoughts of the radiologist quoted at the beginning of this chapter, J. H. E. wrote:

> I would suggest that the practice of radiography by laymen be made a penal offence, and that laws be passed which will render it impossible for the practice of radiography to be carried out by other than skilled and trained medical experts.

Realistically, once it became clear that the radiologists could no longer stake a real claim to monopolise the process of producing X-ray images, their attention turned towards regulating those individuals who did perform this task. In his 1919 paper 'The place of the radiologist and his kindred in the world of medicine', F. Hernaman-Johnson outlined his thoughts on the differences between radiologists and (who would become) radiographers. With regard to the latter he felt it appropriate . . .

> To organise and educate the various classes of lay helpers. To see that their status, remuneration and prospects are such as to make them contented.
> To educate the public as to why such people are at one and the same time invaluable as helpers, and extraordinarily dangerous when they seek to practise independently.

Whatever his motives, Hernaman-Johnson had outlined the basis of a new profession and its underpinning with the concepts of appropriate education and quality control. He did, however, end his paper by returning to a recurring theme:

We should welcome lay assistance, and seek to organize and guide it. It is too late in the day to make a mystery of taking plates but the interpretation is ours for ever.

Hernaman-Johnson was subsequently instrumental in the formation of the Society of Radiographers (and its incorporation in 1920). The Society itself (admittedly with an overwhelming medical presence on its Council) immediately set about the process of establishing the definitive roles of radiologist and radiographer once and for all. In April 1924 a resolution was made by the Council that:

> The membership of the Society of Radiographers does not imply that the member is in possession of the necessary medical knowledge or training for the giving of diagnostic reports and that the responsibility for the diagnosis must rest with the medical man in charge of the case.

During the next 20 years, despite strong opposition from a small number of radiographers, the concept of non-medical staff reporting X-ray films became essentially obsolete. In 1944, C. W. Furby (a radiographer) stated that:

> The primary function of the radiographer is to be of utmost service to the radiologist. The function of the radiologist is the interpretation of the radiograph.

It was not until 1971 that the debate really opened again. Swinburne, a radiologist, writing in *The Lancet*, proposed that radiographers could be used to distinguish between normal and abnormal films. He justified this suggestion on two grounds: (i) 'the chronic shortage of radiologists', and (ii) the fact that radiographers seemed to function below their full potential. These two themes have caused considerable debate since that time. As radiologists are we:

- cynically using strategies to cope with increased radiological workload by getting someone else to help with the work? Or
- altruistically developing skills in fellow professionals and thus enhancing job satisfaction for our radiographer colleagues?

As in many things, the answer probably lies somewhere between the two extremes. It is clear, however, that if the former is the case, many motivated radiographers view it as a reasonable price to pay in order to achieve the latter. Swinburne's paper also touched on several other areas that have been central to the debate. He felt that if radiographers' skills were developed it would improve recruitment and lead to graduate-level careers.

Over the next 20 years the radiological and medical literature featured several publications which made it clear that not only were a relatively small proportion of radiographic examinations actually being reported, but that there was much debate within the medical community as to whether it was even appropriate for a radiologist to attempt to report every image. Against this background, radiographers performing obstetric ultrasound scanning were beginning to provide reports to their medical colleagues. Initially these reports were in the form of numerical data but, gradually, statements of a more interpretational nature were being formulated. This change of emphasis was brought about by demand from the obstetricians. The College of Radiographers responded to this in 1988 by amending the Code of Professional Conduct to state that 'a radiographer may provide a description of images, measurements and numerical data, especially in medical ultrasound'. By 1994 the Code of Conduct stated that 'Radiographers may provide a verbal comment on image appearance to the patient, and should provide a written report to the referring clinician'.

In 1987, Cheyne *et al.* in the paper 'The radiographer and frontline diagnosis' introduced the concept of the 'red dot' system. This system has gone some way to formalising the informal verbal discussions that take place between radiographers and junior doctors (particularly casualty officers) in X-ray departments the world over. It also provides a relatively comfortable halfway house between reporting and non-reporting radiographers.

Pulling these threads together in an editorial in *Clinical Radiology* in 1992, Hugh Saxton, addressing the problems of radiological workload and unreported films, stated that:

> Turning to the field of interpretation, there is little doubt that with careful training suitable radiographers could undertake reporting in such areas as mammography screening or fracture reporting on accident and emergency films.

Having spent nearly 100 years preventing non-medical staff from reporting radiographs, the radiological profession was beginning to come around to the idea.

The early 1990s saw a twin-pronged approach from both district general hospital and teaching hospital backgrounds. In 1994 Loughran published an account of an in-house training scheme in trauma radiology for a group of radiographers and its subsequent assessment. The latter confirmed Saxton's predictions by documenting levels of diagnostic accuracy for the radiographers comparable to the accepted 'gold standards'. In 1995, the results of the Extended Role of the Radiographer project were published. This was a joint enterprise between the Leeds College of Health and St. James' University Hospital (with financial backing from the Department of Health) involving radiographer reporting of trauma, chest and abdomen films. Once again, it became clear that suitably trained radiographers could report X-rays to a high standard.

The final piece in the jigsaw was the publication of the Audit Commission report *Improving Your Image* in 1995. This document, which attempted to address the growing problem of radiological workload, had a number of controversial elements (including advocating the implementation of widespread 'hot reporting'), but its suggestion that radiographers could be used to fill the shortfall in reporting services provoked little response in the radiological literature.

From this point it was clear that not only was there a perceived and documented need for radiographers to contribute to the spiralling radiological workload, but there was also an evidence base confirming that, appropriately trained, they could perform this role to a high standard. The debate had moved on from 'Should they do it?' to 'Could they do it?'. Was there actually a large enough cohort of radiographers able and willing to take on this extended role? The next step involved the development of postgraduate trauma film reporting courses – the lead being taken by Canterbury Christ Church College, and the universities of Bradford, Hertfordshire, Salford and South Bank. These courses were a joint venture between university staff, clinical radiographers, radiography business managers and a group of radiologists who were committed to extending the roles of radiographers in the future.

At the University of Salford, our first cohort of radiographers included two from Macclesfield (whose previous training had been documented in Chris Loughran's paper), two from my own hospital (experienced radiographers who had a particular interest in casualty and orthopaedic radiography), and two from a local children's hospital (underpinning the fact that all the postgraduate courses have paediatric as well as adult elements). The course was accredited by the College of Radiographers relatively easily, following ground-breaking work by Canterbury Christ Church. After this group had graduated, we were keen to assess their abilities objectively. Our study (presented at the UK Radiological Congress in Birmingham in 1999) confirmed that, using a standard set of trauma films, the first group we had trained were significantly better than second-year specialist registrars in radiology, and non-significantly better than third-year specialist registrars.

I have no personal doubt that the traditional boundaries between different professional groups are no longer appropriate in the setting of twenty-first century health care. I have no real problem with any individual (whatever their background) performing any particular task within medicine, as long as they have ability and motivation, are appropriately trained and have a mechanism of audit and risk management in place. I certainly have fewer concerns about the radiographers we have trained than I do about the idea of 'one week' ultrasound courses for general practitioners. It is also a little ironic to start hearing the 'Over my dead body' quote coming from senior radiographers as their junior colleagues try to blur the boundaries further by enrolling on trauma, intravenous urogram (IVU), chest X-ray, computed tomography and gastrointestinal reporting courses. Despite 100 years of history, it is also interesting to note the reaction of some of the radiographic establishment to the fact that other non-medical professionals (notably nurses and physiotherapists) also wish to contribute to patient care by reporting selected imaging techniques. Experience among this text's editors is that 'red dot' courses are becomingly increasingly popular and also increasingly diverse in terms of the professional groups represented on them.

Three other areas deserve consideration from the radiologist's perspective in the context of non-medical staff reporting imaging examina-

Two

tions. The first of these is the impact on radiologist training. The increasing complexity and quantity of radiological work have led to an attempt to ultimately increase the number of consultant radiologists in post by increasing the number of trainees on the training schemes. While this is laudable in itself, it is clear that established consultants, who are already badly stretched, are being asked to increase the amount of time they spend training juniors. The junior radiologists themselves have shown concern that a significant number of consultants are devoting time to training radiographers rather than their own specialist registrars. There may be some perceived merit in the former, as most trained reporting radiographers will stay in their original departments rather than moving elsewhere (unlike specialist registrars). In my view, reporting radiographers can act as a valuable resource in the teaching process rather than a threat – there is no reason why specialist registrars in radiology should not receive basic training in barium enema technique, plain film reporting or IVU management from radiographers.

The second area of concern relates to the shortfall in the number of radiography students coming through the system. The concept of radiographers contributing to areas of work traditionally carried out by radiologists begins to suffer if the radiographers themselves are then not able to 'cover all the bases'. Although radiography is now an established degree-based professional pathway, there is intense competition for enrolment of high quality students. Ironically, although the ultimate 'carrot' of role extension may attract students on to the courses, it only exacerbates the problem if these students are not subsequently interested in the idea of taking the plain films they want to report on. Again, there are echoes of the 1900s in this situation – a split between those who produce the images and those who report them, but this time within the same professional group. It is becomingly increasingly clear that if we are to offer an attractive degree-based professional training with subsequent progression into areas that were previously not part of radiography's remit, there will be 'gaps' which may have to be covered by assistant practitioners or radiography helpers. The radiographic establishment needs to be as open minded about this prospect as it has been about radiographer role extension.

The third area for consideration involves maintaining the heterogeneity of the radiographic profession. I am proud to have been associated with the multi-disciplinary Special Interest Group in Radiographic Reporting, and continue to do all I can to advance the cause of radiographer role extension. I am, however, aware of the fact that there is a large body of dedicated (and often very experienced) radiographers who take great pride in plain film radiography and coping with the demands of providing a plain film service to orthopaedic and casualty departments. Although I can empathise with the statement by the College of Radiographers that 'Reporting by radiographers is not an option for the future, it is a requirement', I feel that it is imperative that those radiographers who do not want to report (but contribute hugely in other ways) are not only allowed to do so but are also positively encouraged, as high professional standards need to be maintained at all levels if we are to provide the optimum service for our patients. Grading and remuneration issues affect both those who want to extend their role and those who don't.

The report and reporting

Having set out the historical context and why it is entirely appropriate for non-medical professionals to report plain films (and other imaging examinations), I would now like to outline my views on how they should go about it by asking (and answering) a few basic questions and outlining some basic principles.

Why are we reporting, and what is a report?

Whatever we are reporting on, whether it be plain film examinations, barium enemas or mammograms, we are commenting on investigations (or 'tests'). The basic reason for performing any investigation is to alter the patient's management – either by providing the definitive diagnosis or by allowing the correct decision to be made about appropriate further treatment. Quite simply, if an investigation cannot potentially do either of these things then it should not be performed – in terms of Ionising Radiation (Medical Exposure) Regulations, it is not clinically justified. By providing a report, we are actually taking part in the clinical decision-making process whereby the result of a 'test' or 'investigation' allows a decision about the patient's management to be made. For example, if we report a fracture it is treated by internal or external fixation; if we report pneumonia it is treated by antibiotics; if we see a tumour it could be treated by excision, while the presence of no abnormality (particularly on trauma films) can mean reassurance or the implementation of conservative therapy. A 'report', therefore, is any form of words or pictures (including a 'red dot') which enables this decision-making process to occur. Ideally, a report should turn a test result into an action.

What constitutes a report?

A report can be entirely based on verbal communication – a direct discussion with the referring clinician face-to-face, by telephone or by an intermediary (an accompanying nurse or even the patient themselves). A provisional (unverified) report can be written in the patient's notes or on a casualty card. The definitive report appears as printed words on a standard form or within a computer screen or field. Verification is an important part of making a report legally binding. Many reporting radiographers type their own reports directly into the departmental computer system. Those reporters who have the luxury of having their reports typed by others need to make an effort to ensure there are no typographical or transcription errors. Remember as well that there may be more than one report in existence, as junior and senior medical staff often document their own interpretation of the images by writing in the case notes.

When is a report not a report?

If we consider an upper abdominal ultrasound examination, the report could be any of the following.

Normal examination.
No abnormality identified.
Normal liver, kidneys, spleen, gall bladder, bile ducts and pancreas.

Although all three versions are factually correct, it may be argued that the last version may be of greatest value to someone who is asked to review the right kidney two years later. They could feel confident that the previous examiner had definitely looked at the organ and felt it to be normal. Furthermore, like the rest of us, clinicians change their minds. The original request card may have stated '? Right renal colic' but two days later, they now feel it is biliary in origin. Did your colleague who wrote statement one actually look at the gall bladder as well or not? Unfortunately, they are now on annual leave, so that you have no option but to repeat the scan. In summary, all three are reports but some forms of report are more useful than others. We need to be aware, however, that the line must be drawn somewhere – what about the aorta, inferior vena cava and adrenals?

What's in a report?

Following on from the last question, and with particular reference to trauma films, we have to make clear decisions about what we are going to include in our reports. How are we going to deal with the presence of old fractures, osteoarthritis, vascular calcification and accessory ossicles? There is no clear answer to this question, although it may be reasonable to mention these features if they are either (i) likely to cause confusion if they are interpreted incorrectly by other staff (accessory ossicles) or (ii) unexpected in a patient of a particular age (premature osteoarthritis or vascular calcification).

The importance of examination technique

Trauma films can be the most difficult to obtain, as patients are either unable (because of pain) or unwilling (because of alcohol or drugs) to co-operate in producing optimum images. There are two points to be made here.

(1) You can't report on what you can't see – if it has not been included on the film, the information is lost.

(2) Trauma film reporting radiographers soon become highly critical of their colleagues' attempts to produce satisfactory images. For most reporting radiographers it is the first time in their careers that they have thought analytically about what is actually on the films and how the images are presented. Do not be too hard on your non-reporting colleagues!

Principles of reporting

The following principles may be worth considering as you approach trauma film reporting.

You can't report on what you can't see: As already mentioned, you can only comment on what is included in the film. If the radiograph does not cover the whole area of interest you may wish to document the fact.

Look at everything on the film: You may be the only one who does. It is easy for the eye to get drawn to an area of obvious abnormality, resulting in a less than comprehensive review of the rest of the film. Look at all the bone and soft tissue outlines – secondary or associated injuries are not uncommon. On occasions (for example, the presence of soft tissue swelling over the lateral malleolus, or the presence of an elbow fat pad sign) there may be significant injury in the presence of normal bony outlines.

Be thorough to the point of obsession: Work your way systematically around all the cortical bone of hand and foot views. Experienced clinicians who 'immediately' spot the fractured phalanx still have to review the rest of the radiograph.

Learn to love your 'bright light': There are still a large number of clinicians (junior and not so junior) who don't realise that the 'black' bits of the radiograph still contain valuable information if bright-lighted. Do, however, spare a thought for the junior doctors working in the average casualty department. It is often hard enough for them to find a viewing box, let alone a bright light or quiet spot to systematically analyse the film.

Although you should bear in mind my previous point about 'when is a report not a report', it is generally not advisable to make your reports too long. The people who are going to read your report have a short attention span and many distractions.

Don't sit on the fence: 'Defensive' reporting may or may not have its place, but the whole point of trauma film reporting is to help manage the patient sitting in the casualty department. As you gain experience and become established, the clinicians you work with will come to rely on your reports. They will appreciate that there will be occasions where you make a mistake, but they are basically asking you to answer a relatively straightforward question. By all means use your words carefully, but don't leave any doubt as to whether you think the film is abnormal or not.

Film viewing

As you sit down to report your pile of trauma films you should consider the following.

- Sit comfortably – you need to concentrate on the film not your chair.
- Try to report in a (relatively) quiet, darkened room or area – maximise your ability to see abnormalities.
- Use an appropriate masking device – most casualty films are small, and masking areas of the viewing box not needed to display the film will effectively improve the viewing conditions.
- If appropriate (for example, scaphoid follow-ups) try to ensure that you have the previous films for comparison purposes.
- Read the clinical information. It may well only say '?#', but it may be useful in localising the abnormality and, on occasion, allows minor cortical irregularities to be consigned to the 'not worth mentioning' part of your brain if they are on the non-symptomatic side of the hand, foot or skull.
- Assess the technical quality of the film. As I have already mentioned, try not to be too critical of your colleague who has performed the examination – it may have been a demanding and difficult patient. There is, however, a place for constructive criticism, as you know precisely what you were looking for on the film, and whether it was demonstrated or not.
- After taking a general overview of the film, pass on to closer systematic inspection (using a bright light or magnifying glass as needed). You then need to apply the three Ds.

The three Ds

There are many published systems of film analysis for casualty and other radiographs. I find the three Ds useful as a framework.

- Describe – may be enough in most normal films.
- Diagnose – is there a fracture? If so, what is it? Are there other associated abnormalities?
- Direct – further views or investigations may be needed.

Standard phrases

Having assessed the film, you will start the process of formulating a report and transferring it to tape or inputting it via a computer keyboard. At this point you may wish to make use of a bank of standard phrases available to you.

- No fracture.
- No fracture seen.
- No acute fracture seen.
- Normal bony and soft tissue outlines.
- There is soft tissue swelling overlying the (lateral malleolus), but no fracture can be seen.
- If clinical suspicion of scaphoid fracture persists, repeat views in 7–10 days time are recommended.

Remember that most examinations are essentially normal. If there is an abnormality present, you will need to have a similar bank of phrases to describe it. Think about how your different radiological and radiographic colleagues describe abnormalities. What are their favourite phrases? Be prepared to 'cut and paste' their reporting styles as you develop your own.

Communication

Reporting is about communication. Different clinicians require different degrees of communication (and you can read that any way you like!). Learn what your clinicians want from your reports – remember they are your customers. While the customer may always be right, remember that you can't please everybody all the time. Develop a style that is the 'best fit' for the group of clinicians you work with.

If you are going to communicate effectively and efficiently with your clinicians, you need to be able to talk their language. To this end you should take any opportunity you have to attend fracture clinics, orthopaedic clinics and relevant clinico-radiological meetings. If you use a scoring system in any aspect of your reporting, make sure that everyone (including the locum senior house officer) knows exactly what you mean by it.

What if I get it wrong?

The medico-legal aspects of reporting are covered elsewhere in this book. However, I know that this is an area that non-medical reporting practitioners find particularly worrying. In the case of radiographers, part of the problem lies in taking the big step from a mistake which results in consigning a film to the reject drawer to a reporting error which adversely affects the wellbeing of a patient. Somewhere during their

Two

Two

training, doctors seem to have come to terms with the fact that they will, inevitably, make mistakes during their careers. Clearly nobody likes to make a mistake, but if your day-to-day practice is of a high standard, then that is how you will be judged by your colleagues. Reporting protocols are widely available and, as far as I am concerned, ratification by the trust board of the actions of appropriately qualified radiographers working within agreed guidelines clearly implies where legal culpability lies.

Conclusion

I have outlined a radiologist's perspective of non-medical practitioners reporting trauma films. I have briefly outlined the historical process of 'should they' and 'could they'. I have also tried to analyse exactly what a report is, its role in the decision-making process, and outlined a brief plan to facilitate film analysis and report composition. I have also made some brief (and very personal) comments on what happens when we get it wrong. I think I can do no better in summarising than to quote Lewis Carroll:

> 'Then you should say what you mean,' the March Hare went on.
> 'I do,' Alice hastily replied; 'at least – at least I mean what I say – that's the same thing you know.'
> 'Not the same thing a bit!' said the Hatter.

The essence of successful trauma film reporting is to say what you mean **and** mean what you say.

Acknowledgement

I would like to acknowledge Richard Price of the University of Hertfordshire, whose excellent and informative paper 'Radiographer reporting: origins, demise and revival of plain film reporting' (*Radiography*, 2001, 7, 105–17) was the source of several of the references in the section on the history of reporting.

3 Legal Aspects Arising in the Reporting of X-rays

Professor Bridget Dimond

Introduction

Reporting by radiographers is now well established in the UK as Professor Thomas in Chapter 2 of this book illustrates. It is the intention of this chapter to describe briefly the legal context within which a range of practitioners perform a reporting function. The chapter will then demonstrate the kinds of legal questions that arise and, through examples, outline the main laws that apply. A list of further reading is provided so that the reader can follow up in more details the topics that will be discussed[1].

Legal system

Laws derive from two main sources: first, acts of Parliament (known as primary legislation) and regulations (known as secondary legislation) or laws, directions or regulations from the European Community and, second, the decisions in cases decided by the courts (known as the common law, judge made law or case law). The assemblies of Scotland, Wales and Northern Ireland have varying law-making powers. Primary legislation often gives powers to a minister of the Crown to make further, more detailed regulations. These are usually drawn up in the form of a statutory instrument, which is laid before Parliament for approval or rejection before it comes into force.

Human Rights Act

This Act came into force on 2 October 2000 (in Scotland on devolution) and has three effects.

Three

- All public authorities or organisations carrying out functions of a public nature are required to respect the European Convention of Human Rights which is set out in Schedule 1 of the Act.
- Citizens have a right to bring an action in the courts of the UK if they consider that their human rights, as set out in the Schedule, had been breached by a public authority.
- Judges are required to refer back to Parliament any legislation that they consider to be incompatible with the articles set out in the European Convention of Human Rights.

One of the most significant changes brought about by this Act is that people no longer have to take their case to Strasbourg for a hearing before the European Court of Human Rights but can avoid the additional cost and delay and bring the case before UK courts. If a judicial review is sought of a decision that is considered to be in breach of the human rights recognised in the Convention, then legal aid is available for this action.

Of specific significance to the health professional are the following articles:

- Article 2 – the right to life;
- Article 3 – the right not to be subjected to torture or to inhuman or degrading treatment and punishment;
- Article 5 – the right to liberty and security of person;
- Article 6 – the right to fair and independent hearings;
- Article 8 – the right to respect for private and family life, home and correspondence;
- Article 9 – the right of respect for religion, belief, etc;
- Article 10 – the right of freedom of expression;
- Article 14 – the right not to be discriminated against in the recognition of the articles.

The articles can be downloaded from the internet from the website of the Department of Health[2]. It is possible that a patient could argue that he or she was treated in an inhuman and degrading way (so breaching Article 3) because their X-ray examination was reported upon by a radiographer who failed to identify an abnormality.

The legality of the delegation of reporting

Unless there is a statute which expressly requires a specific activity to be carried out by a person registered with a particular health profession, then anyone can undertake that activity provided that they have the competence, knowledge, experience, expertise and supervision to enable it to be done at the same reasonable standard of care that the professional who would ordinarily have done that activity would have followed

---

Box 3.1   Delegation of specified medical activity.

The Royal College of Nurses (RCN) queried the legality of the practice where nurses supervised patients who were undergoing termination of pregnancies by prostaglandin in the light of the wording of the Abortion Act 1969 that the pregnancy should be terminated by a registered medical practitioner. The RCN brought a case on behalf of its members against the Department of Health and Social Security (DHSS) because members had complained that they were often left on wards to supervise (sometimes for several days) a patient who was having a prostaglandin-induced abortion. The doctor would set up the drip and then the nurse would undertake the care of the patient. The RCN questioned, in particular, advice given in a DHSS letter and circular relating to the procedures that might be performed by an appropriately skilled nurse or midwife[3].

Box 3.2   Lord Diplock's view in the case of *Royal College of Nursing* v *The Department of Health and Social Security* 1981 1 All ER 545.

'In the context of the Act what was required was that a registered medical practitioner – a doctor – should accept responsibility for all stages of the treatment for the termination of the pregnancy. The particular method to be used should be decided by the doctor in charge of that treatment; he should carry out any physical acts, forming part of the treatment, that in accordance with accepted medical practice were done only by qualified medical practitioners, and should give specific instructions as to the carrying out of such parts of the treatment as in accordance with accepted medical practice were carried out by nurses or other hospital staff without medical qualifications. To each of them the doctor or his substitute should be available to be consulted or called in for assistance from beginning to end of the treatment. In other words, the doctor need not do everything with his own hands; the subsection's requirements were satisfied when the treatment was one prescribed by a registered medical practitioner carried out in accordance with his directions and of which he remained in charge throughout.'

Three

(see discussion of standards below). However, even where a statute specifically requires a particular health professional to undertake the activity, the House of Lords has held that there is compliance with the statute if another person undertakes that activity under the supervision of the specified health professional. This decision was made in relation to the Abortion Act 1969. The facts of the case are shown in Box 3.1 and the justification for the majority decision of the House of Lords as stated by Lord Diplock in Box 3.2.

The House of Lords decided on a majority of three to two that the DHSS advice did not involve the performance of unlawful acts by members of the RCN. Lord Diplock's views are set out in Box 3.2.

There are no statutory provisions that would prevent the activity of reporting on X-rays being delegated to non-medical staff.

Standards of practice

Common law, however, requires that where activities are delegated, the patient is entitled to receive the same standard of care that could have been expected had the activity not been delegated. The test for what would be a reasonable standard of care was laid down in a case in 1957 involving the administration of electroconvulsive therapy (ECT) to a patient[4]. The courts use what has now become known as Bolam's test. In the Bolam case Judge McNair said:

> The standard of care expected is the standard of the ordinary skilled man exercising and professing to have that special skill.

Case law has also established that even an inexperienced person is expected to provide the reasonable standard of care as the case in Box 3.3 illustrates.

The crucial question in the case was: since Mrs Weston was not a qualified driver, was the standard of care that she owed to Mr Nettleship lower than would otherwise have been the case? The court decided not. They preferred to have one standard of driving, not a variable standard depending on the characteristics of the individual driver:

> The certainty of a general standard is preferable to the vagaries of a fluctuating standard.
>
> (Lord Justice Megaw)

Lord Justice Megaw, in discussing the issue, used the example of the young surgeon:

> Suppose that to the knowledge of the patient, a young surgeon, whom the patient has chosen to operate on him, has only just qualified. If the operation goes wrong because of the surgeon's inexperience, is there a defence on the basis that the standard of care and skill was lower than the standard of a competent and experienced surgeon? In cases such as the present it is preferable that there should be a reasonably certain and reasonably ascertainable standard of care, even if on occasion that may appear to work hardly against an inexperienced driver.

(Mr Nettleship obtained his compensation, subject to a reduction for contributory negligence.)

Box 3.3   An inexperienced driver.

Mr Nettleship was teaching Mrs Weston to drive in her husband's car. On the third lesson he was helping her by moving the gear lever, applying the hand-brake and occasionally helping with the steering. In the course of the lesson they made a slow left-hand turn after stopping at a halt sign. However, Mrs Weston did not straighten up the wheel and panicked. Mr Nettleship got hold of the handbrake with one hand and tried to get hold of the steering wheel with the other. The car hit a lamp standard. Mr Nettleship broke his knee-cap. He claimed compensation and succeeded before the Court of Appeal[5].

The Court of Appeal in a more recent case has stated that a junior practitioner will be expected to provide the reasonable standard of care which a more senior person would provide[6]. Clearly there are responsibilities upon senior staff and managers to ensure that the reasonable standard of care for the patient is provided. The Court of Appeal also held that the courts do not recognise the existence of team liability. Each individual practitioner is personally and professionally accountable for his or her own actions and cannot blame the team or team instructions for negligence that has led to harm.

It follows, therefore, that if a radiographer who had undertaken reporting activities missed an abnormality which a radiologist would have noticed, it would be no defence to an action brought by the patient who had suffered harm as a consequence that it was a radiographer who reported on the film and not a radiologist. In practice, as Professor Thomas has shown in Chapter 2 (p. 11), monitoring would suggest that there is a very high standard of reporting by radiographers measured against second- and third-year specialist registrars in radiology. All the points that he makes about the standards of the actual report should be part of the training of the radiographer, so ensuring that there are clear professional standards on what a satisfactory report should or should not contain.

Safe expansion of the radiographer's role

The *NHS Plan*[7] envisages that other professionals could undertake many activities at present undertaken by medical staff. No changes in legisla-

---

Box 3.4   Principles for adjusting the scope of professional practice.

The health professional:

- must be satisfied that each aspect of practice is directed to meeting the needs and serving the interests of the patient or client;
- must endeavour always to achieve, maintain and develop knowledge, skill and competence to respond to those needs and interests;
- must honestly acknowledge any limits of personal knowledge and skill and take steps to remedy any relevant deficits in order effectively and appropriately to meet the needs of patients and clients;
- must ensure that any enlargement or adjustment of the scope of personal professional practice must be achieved without compromising or fragmenting existing aspects of professional practice and care and that requirements of the council's code of professional conduct are satisfied throughout the whole area of practice;
- must recognise and honour the direct or indirect personal accountability borne for all aspects of professional practice; and
- must, in serving the interests of patients and clients and the wider interests of society, avoid any inappropriate delegation to others which compromises those interests.

tion would be necessary. Where particular professions have been identified in law (as in the Medicines Act and the Misuse of Drugs Act) then amending legislation has been enacted. In order to ensure that standards are maintained, where activities are delegated careful preparation is necessary for other professions to take over these activities. The United Kingdom Central Council for Nursing, Midwifery and Health Visiting (now superseded by the Nursing and Midwifery Council) published *Scope of Professional Practice*[8], a document that set out the principles to guide the safe development of professional practice. While the document itself has since been superseded by the *Code of Professional Practice*[9] the principles still remain relevant to professions other than nursing and are shown in Box 3.4.

Can a radiographer refuse to undertake reporting on films?

Professor Thomas in Chapter 2 states:

> . . . it is imperative that those radiographers who do not want to report (but contribute hugely in other ways) are not only allowed to do so, but are positively encouraged, as high professional standards need to be maintained at all levels if we are to provide the optimum service for our patients.

It was certainly a principle under the concept of the 'extended role of the nurse' that a nurse could refuse to undertake a new task or activity[10]. It probably no longer applies to the registered nurse and one could question whether this principle of refusal is still appropriate in relation to the scope of professional practice of the radiographer. All health professionals registered with the Health Professions Council (HPC) have a duty to maintain and improve their professional knowledge and competence. Although the HPC has not yet introduced professional development criteria for re-registration it has indicated its intention to do so. At the time of writing the HPC has decided that continuing professional development (CPD) will be linked to registration, but it will not come into effect for at least three years. The HPC has, however, decided to hold another consultation on this within two years when it will set out its proposals in more detail. It has already decided, however, that CPD should:

- avoid monitoring registrants' compliance based simply on the number of hours undertaken each year;
- be linked to national standards;
- take account of the work of others, such as the Allied Health Professions' (AHP) project on demonstrating competence through CPD that is already being undertaken;

- take account of the needs of part-time and self-employed registrants; and
- require individual registrants to commit themselves to CPD.

It would seem to be entirely inappropriate for a practitioner to refuse to develop his or her professional practice beyond the level he or she reached at registration. As the role of the radiographer expands, reporting may become a more significant part of that role. Clearly the radiographer would be contractually entitled to receive from the employer the necessary training to ensure that he or she was competent in the new range of activities. It is a contractual requirement of the employer to ensure that staff are competent to undertake the work that they are asked to perform. There are other contractual considerations. In an interview for a job, for example, a radiographer might be told that a contractual requirement for that particular post is that the radiographer is able to report on specific radiographs. If the radiographer agrees to this condition of employment then he or she is contractually bound to develop, with support from the employer, the appropriate skills, knowledge and competence. If the interviewee refuses the condition, they will probably not get the post.

In applying the law to the situation of Bob Smith in Box 3.5 it could be said that Bob has not agreed at his interview to undertake reporting. However, there is an implied term in the contract of employment that employees have a duty to obey reasonable instructions of the employer. Is it a reasonable instruction for Bob to be asked to develop his scope of professional practice? Much would depend upon the detailed circumstances. Is the training he is being offered reasonable and would he be competent to undertake reporting as a consequence? Would the areas on which he would be expected to report come within what could reasonably be expected of an appropriately trained radiographer? Would there be staff available to undertake the work that he would ordinarily be doing had he not been engaged in reporting? (Clearly to expect staff to undertake an expanded role without at the same time examining their total workload and facilitating some delegation of existing activities would be unreasonable.) Perhaps a radiographer could put forward arguments suggesting that the request to Bob in Box 3.5 is unreasonable at present, but over time it might become a reasonable requirement. The quote from Chapter 2 (pp. 12–13) may well be appropriate at the present time, but there may come a time when reporting is seen as crucial to the role of the radiographer.

Box 3.5 Refusing to report.

There was a serious shortage of radiologists in Roger Park NHS Trust and radiographer Bob Smith was asked by his head of department to go on a training course for plain film chest X-ray reporting. Bob said that had he wished to be a radiologist he would have trained as one and he did not wish to undertake the training. What is the law?

Accountability: criminal, employer's, professional and civil

Could a radiographer be held accountable if a patient were to die as a result of a failure by the radiographer to identify an abnormality? Box 3.6 sets out a situation where a death has occurred following a failure to identify a significant abnormality on a radiograph. This situation will be explored to illustrate the criminal, civil, disciplinary and professional proceedings which could take place.

Coroner

In the case of an unexpected death as in Box 3.6, the death will have to be reported to the coroner. The statutory duty of the coroner is to establish the identity of the deceased, how, where and when the deceased came by their death and the particulars, for the time being required by the Registration Acts, to be registered concerning the death. The coroner cannot make a finding that any person is criminally responsible for the death. However, he or she can adjourn the inquest and ask the police and Crown Prosecution Service to consider criminal proceedings. The third report of the Shipman Inquiry has recommended fundamental changes to the certification of death and the jurisdiction and office of the coroner[11].

Box 3.6   Who is to blame?

Emily (a radiographer) is on duty when Fred (a patient) comes into the department carrying an X-ray request card. Fred had been involved in a road traffic accident and his chest had hit against the wheel of the car. He was not wearing a seat belt. Emily took the radiograph and checked that a further one did not need to be taken, before sending Fred back to Accident and Emergency (A&E). She said that she would send the X-ray through to A&E. The X-ray department used a system of radiographer reporting, and so Emily studied the X-ray and decided that nothing abnormal could be seen. Once the radiograph with Emily's 'No Abnormality Detected (NAD)' note arrived in A&E the junior doctor called for Fred and he was advised that there appeared to be nothing abnormal on the X-ray and he could go home. He was advised to take it very carefully for a few days and to return immediately to the department if he experienced any sharp pain or fainting symptoms. Unfortunately, Fred died six hours after leaving the A&E department. A post-mortem examination showed that he had died of a collapse of a lung which had been punctured. Fred's family have complained about the failure of the hospital to diagnose his condition and have made it clear that they intend to take legal action and obtain compensation. Fred was 45 years of age and earned £50 000 a year. He has a family with three children and his wife is a full-time mother and housewife.

Criminal proceedings

Health professionals can be found guilty of manslaughter if they have acted with such gross negligence in carrying out their professional work that their actions amount to a criminal act. This was the ruling by the House of Lords in the case of *R.* v *Adomako*[12] where an anaesthetist was held guilty of manslaughter after a patient had died on the operating table. A doctor in Nottingham pleaded guilty to manslaughter as a result of his gross negligence after administering a chemotherapeutic drug by epidural rather than intravenous injection which led to the death of a patient suffering from leukaemia. He was given a prison sentence. In contrast, the prosecution of two surgeons from Prince Phillip Hospital, Llanelly, for manslaughter, when they removed the wrong kidney, failed since the prosecution were unable to show that removal of the wrong kidney caused the death of the patient. The jury were ordered to bring forward a verdict acquitting the doctors. In the situation in Box 3.6 it would have to be established that failure to identify the abnormality in Fred's condition was gross professional negligence by Emily, the junior doctor in A&E or some other person who was caring for Fred and that this gross negligence caused the death of Fred.

Disciplinary proceedings

The employer of the person whose actions have caused harm would be entitled to take disciplinary action against the employee. There is an implied term in a contract of employment that an employee will act with reasonable care and skill and obey reasonable instructions. An investigation would have to take place and if it was established that the radiographer and/or the A&E junior doctor failed to make the appropriate diagnosis or follow the correct procedure, steps within the disciplinary procedure from an oral warning to dismissal on the ground of gross misconduct could take place.

Professional conduct proceedings

Any registered health professional would also face professional conduct proceedings that could lead to them being struck off the register. The actions of a radiographer would be reported to the HPC which has the power to investigate the situation and, if considered appropriate, to hold a conduct and competence hearing. Similar professional conduct proceedings can be held by the General Medical Council in respect of the A&E junior doctor.

Civil proceedings

All health professionals owe a duty of care to their patients. If a patient has suffered harm as a result of negligence by a health professional then the patient could bring an action for negligence against that person or, more usually, the employer of that person. The latter action is possible because of the doctrine of vicarious liability that makes the employer liable for any harm caused by the negligence of an employee who was acting in the course of his or her employment. Any claimant would have to show that the employee owed a duty of care that was broken when the employee failed to follow a reasonable standard of care that caused the reasonably foreseeable harm. To determine if there has been a breach of the duty of care, the courts have used Bolam's test[4], which has been discussed above.

If these elements of duty, breach, causation and harm can be established, then compensation is payable to the claimant. In the case of a death, there is a fixed statutory sum payable to the estate of the deceased (at present £10 000) but, in addition, those persons who were dependent upon the deceased, for example wife and children, can claim in respect of their loss. In Fred's situation in Box 3.6 (p. 26) there is clearly a duty of care owed to Fred, but has there been a breach of duty and if so, by whom and did this breach of duty cause the death of Fred? In particular, what is the standard of care expected of the radiographer and is Emily accountable for her failure?

Is a reporting radiographer accountable for the reporting?

This may appear to be a strange question to put but the suggestion was made at a conference at the University of Hertfordshire that although a radiographer could assist a doctor by using the 'red dot' system, failure by the radiographer to identify an abnormality should not lead to any repercussions and the radiographer should not be accountable for such a failure. The discussion led the author to write an article about accountability by a radiographer for reporting[13].

It would appear in practice that unless a doctor can rely upon a report by a radiographer being accurate, the doctor must make sure that he or she takes time to examine the film and ignores a 'nothing abnormal' report from the radiographer. If a red dot system is used and there is no red dot, does this mean that there is, on an immediate assessment of the image, no obvious abnormality, i.e. NAD? Alternatively, does it mean that the radiographer has negligently failed to spot an evident abnormality but will not be held accountable for this omission, since the junior doctor or nurse will be the accountable professional? If the doctor can place no reliance upon a reasonable standard of care by the radiographer, it may be wiser not to have a red dot or reporting system involving a radiographer. The doctor needs to be assured that if a red dot system is operating, those undertaking it will follow the reasonable standard of care of a qualified and trained radiographer in making an assessment. There would appear to be no justification in law for holding that a health professional who is undertaking a delegated activity is not accountable for his or her practice. It would be contrary to all the basic principles of the law to exempt a registered professional from the legal effects of negligence.

In the joint paper published by the Royal College of Radiologists and the Society and College of Radiographers in defining the two elements of reporting, the descriptive report and the medical report, it is stated that the descriptive report may be provided by those members of the team who are competent to do so, in accordance with a protocol agreed by the medical members of the team[14]. The author of the descriptive report bears responsibility for its content. The medical report provides a report and opinion on the further medical management of the patient and this can be provided only by an appropriately trained registered medical practitioner, normally a radiologist. This would appear to be a reasonable approach and certainly recognises the responsibility of the radiographer providing the descriptive report.

Applying the law to the situation in Box 3.6 (p. 26), if any reasonable radiographer trained to report would have identified the abnormality in Fred's film, then Emily is in breach of her duty of care and negligent. If, however, it was not an abnormality that could easily have been identified in a film then there is no breach of the duty of care, for further discussion on abnormality detection see p. 35. However, to obtain compensation under our present system of civil claims for clinical negligence, the claimant must also establish that the breach of duty caused the harm. If Emily has been negligent, whether or not her negligence caused the harm depends upon what the appropriate system for safeguarding patients should be. Should there have been a follow-up report by a radiologist that would have identified Fred's condition in time to save his life? If the answer is that there should have been such a system and this would have identified his condition, then there is negligence by the NHS trust in failing to set up the appropriate system for patient care. If the answer is that such a system was not necessary and it was reasonable practice to rely upon the report of the radiographer, then Emily's negligence would appear to have led to the death of Fred, in which case (and if appropriate action could have been taken to save Fred's life, had his condition been correctly diagnosed) her employers would be vicariously liable to his family.

Future changes in compensation for clinical negligence

The Department of Health has recently published a consultation paper recommending the introduction of an NHS Redress Scheme[15] that would provide a new statutory scheme for claiming compensation for clinical negligence. One important feature of the scheme is that potential claims should, in the early stages, be handled as part of the complaints system.

Conclusions

The College of Radiographers in its vision paper states that[16]:

> Reporting by radiographers is not an option for the future, it is a requirement.

It is, however, only one of many other activities that may be taken on by a radiographer. For example, the Ionising Radiation (Medical Exposure) Regulations 2000 can be seen as an example of the government recognising the value of flexibility in who does what in the health services. The regulations focus on the responsibilities to be assumed by any competent healthcare professional who undertakes the duties, rather than on the professional background of the person. Thus the definitions of referrer, practitioner and operator all emphasise the competence of the individual to perform that function rather than on a particular professional background.

Prescribing medicines is another area where radiographers are able to practise after appropriate training. Radiographers are one of the named health professionals able to prescribe under Patient Group Directions[17].

The NHS Plan[7] envisages a far more flexible multi-skilled work force. It is essential therefore that reporting by radiographers should not be seen as a short-term solution to the current shortage of radiologists, but should be part of a planned development of the scope of professional practice of the radiographer and the implications for other health professionals, including the use of healthcare support workers in X-ray departments, should be explored. There are many justifications for radiographers to have the additional training, supervision and experience which enables them to develop an expertise in identifying abnormalities in certain radiographs. Equally important is the need to define the parameters of their reporting work so that they can be held professionally and personally accountable for what they do.

References

1   Dimond, B. (2002) *Legal Aspects of Radiography and Radiology.* Blackwell Science, Oxford.
2   Department of Health (2003) website: www.doh.gov.uk/humanrights (accessed November 2003).
3   *Royal College of Nursing* v *Department of Health and Social Security* 1981 1 All ER 545.

4   *Bolam* v *Friern Hospital Management Committee* [1957] 1 WLR 582.
5   *Nettleship* v *Weston* 1971 3 All ER 581.
6   *Wilsher* v *Essex Area Health Authority* [1986] 3 All ER 801.
7   Department of Health (2000) *The NHS Plan*. The Stationery Office, London.
8   United Kingdom Central Council (1992) *The Scope of Professional Practice*. UKCC, London.
9   Nursing and Midwifery Council (2003) *Code of Professional Conduct*. NMC, London.
10 Department of Health *Health Circular HC (77)22*. DoH, London.
11 The Shipman Inquiry Third Report (14 July 2003) *Death and Cremation Certification*. www.the-shipman-inquiry.ortg.uk/reports.asp (accessed November 2003).
12 *Regina* v *Adomako* [1994] 2 All ER 79.
13 Dimond, B. (2000) Red dots and radiographer's liability. *Health Care Risk Report* **6**(10), 10–12.
14 Royal College of Radiologists and Society and College of Radiographers (1998) *Interprofessional Roles and Responsibilities in a Radiology Service*. RCR, London.
15 Department of Health (2003) *Making Amends: a consultation paper setting out proposals for reforming the approach to clinical negligence in the NHS*. CMO, London.
16 College of Radiographers (1997) *Reporting by Radiographers: A Vision Paper*. CoR, London.
17 Department of Health (2000) *Prescription Only Medicines (Human Use)*. SI 2000 No 1917. DoH, London.

Further reading

Dimond, B. (2002) *Legal Aspects of Pain Management*. Quay Publications, Mark Allen Press, Dinton, Salisbury.

Dimond, B. (2002) *Legal Aspects of Patient Confidentiality*. Quay Publications, Mark Allen Press, Dinton, Salisbury.

Dimond, B. (2002) *Legal Aspects of Radiography and Radiology*. Blackwell Science, Oxford.

Dimond, B. (2003) *Legal Aspects of Consent*. Quay Publications, Mark Allen Press, Dinton, Salisbury.

Hurwitz, B. (1998) *Clinical Guidelines and the Law*. Radcliffe Medical Press, Oxford.

Kennedy, I. and Grubb, A. (2000) *Medical Law and Ethics*, 3rd edn. Butterworth, London.

McHale, J. and Tingle, J. (2001) *Law and Nursing*. Butterworth-Heinemann, London.

Pitt, G. (2000) *Employment Law*, 4th edn. Sweet and Maxwell, London.

Selwyn, N. (2000) *Selwyn's Law of Employment*, 11th edn. Butterworth, London.

Wilkinson, R. and Caulfield, H. (2000) *The Human Rights Act: A Practical Guide for Nurses*. Whurr Publishers, London.

Three

4 Uncertainty and Bias in Decision Making

Dr Ian Christensen

Introduction

Human beings usually learn to manage uncertainty in most areas of their lives and we are continually making decisions in order to function in an environment whose behaviour we can only imperfectly predict. However, the fact that we can become very practised at decision making does not mean that we make our decisions in an optimal way. In fact our decisions are frequently biased and the impact of these biases will depend on the domain in which they occur. In many day-to-day circumstances faulty decision making may lead to little more than irritation and minor inconvenience. Other environments are less forgiving, and faulty decisions can have serious consequences.

Interpreting medical images inevitably involves decisions, because we can only examine a **representation** of the state of organs and tissues: we cannot examine them directly. Since the relation between the image and the true state of the tissue under investigation may not always be veridical the clinician will always have to manage a degree of uncertainty about what is 'really' there. This chapter provides an account of psychological concepts and research that have helped us understand how people 'naturally' make decisions in these kinds of circumstances. This understanding can help teachers and practitioners improve their professional performance by helping them to avoid common sources of bias and error.

All types of decision making have certain fundamental elements in common: the gathering and evaluation of evidence, the study of possible outcomes and so on. A psychological analysis may usefully distinguish the importance of three classes or levels of process in which these elements may operate: sensation and perception, individual cognition and social cognition. We routinely make decisions on the basis of the evidence of our senses, and most of the time we are completely unaware that we are in fact making any decision at all. Only when the evidence is ambiguous and the decision is important does the decision making process intrude into consciousness. In this chapter we will deal with one facet of sensory decision making. Other aspects are included in Chapter 5 (Pattern Recognition). The study of individual cognitive processes in decision making covers what most people would recognise as 'proper' decision making. A huge amount has been written on how people *should* make decisions[1] but here we will concern ourselves with some of the psychological factors that can inadvertently introduce error into the process. Finally, when decisions are made by two or more people acting together it is by no means certain that the outcome will be more reliable than that which would be achieved by individuals acting independently. Social processes within a group may interfere with, as well as enhance, dependable decision making.

Sensory decision making: signal detection theory

Signal detection theory deals with decisions that are made purely on the basis of sensory evidence, under conditions where the data are 'noisy' (that is, where the sensory evidence is not clear-cut) and where the decision alternatives are 'yes/no', 'present/absent' or some equivalent binary choice. Decisions like these have often to be made when interpreting images such as skeletal radiographs.

The theory is based on the idea that all sensory observations are made against a background of noise that varies randomly in intensity; when a signal of *fixed* intensity occurs, it is observed against whatever intensity of noise happens to be present at the time. An observer's task is characterised as a decision between two hypotheses: an observation was noise alone, or there was a signal combined *with* the noise. If the signal is larger than the noise then this presents no problem. When it is small, or not there at all, the observer is said to adopt a decision criterion (usually called β) and then make a judgement according to whether the observation exceeds the criterion or not. Observers may decide a signal was present when it was not (a false positive) or miss a signal when it was present (a false negative) as well as correctly saying it was present (true positive) or absent (true negative). Moving the decision criterion will alter the **relative proportions** of the two kinds of mistake but does not improve decision making overall. That is determined by the **discriminability** of the signal (written as **d′**, pronounced 'd prime') from the noise. This theory has been extensively tested and provides an accurate account of how we detect low intensity signals across a variety of sensory modalities. The essential components are illustrated in Figure 4.1.

To illustrate this model in the context of image interpretation, consider the case of a radiographer who has to decide whether a mammogram shows evidence of microcalcification. The 'signal' in this case is the presence of the characteristic tiny white spots on the radiograph. The 'noise' is anything (such as specks of dust) which may mimic the signs, or factors such as poor compression or tissue density that make the film

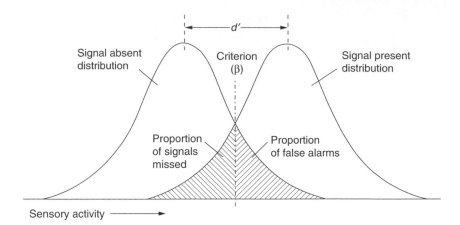

Figure 4.1 The main components of the signal detection theory.

difficult to read. (A second example of noise or the impact of artefact projection onto the image would be the apparent lytic line representing a fracture as in the mach line over the odontoid peg – see Chapter 9, p. 22.) The final decision, let us suppose, is whether to 'red dot' (or abnormality highlight) the film or not. If the evidence is clear (the noise is relatively low-level and the signs are clear) then in terms of Figure 4.1 the observation lies to the right of the decision criterion and the decision is made to red spot the film. If on the other hand there is little sign of microcalcification *relative* to the noise, the observation is to the left of the criterion and the decision is made to pass the film as clear. The effect of changing β is straightforward. Moving it to the right is equivalent to requiring more convincing evidence before making a 'yes' decision. This will reduce the number of false positives, but at the same time increase the number of false negatives, or 'misses'. Moving β to the left will have the reverse effect: there will be more false positives, but fewer misses. The position of β thus has a crucial effect on the outcome of the decision process.

This model also describes the way in which we make many simple day-to-day decisions. Was that the door bell I just heard? Did I just glimpse someone I know in that crowd of people? Although we are not generally aware of how we change our decision criteria, consider how a person might react in the second of those instances. If they would really like to speak to the person they have *perhaps* seen they might make a 'yes' decision and go after them. If they were indifferent about meeting them, or were in too much of a hurry, they might decide 'no' and carry on their way. In fact, research shows[2] that the single most important factor that determines the position of a decision criterion is the **value attached to the outcome**. In either of the mammogram or odontoid peg examples, the radiographer will have to weigh up the relative value of a false alarm (a worried patient is unnecessarily recalled for another test) versus a false negative (the condition may be much worse when it is finally diagnosed correctly). These are complicated judgements to make because in practice it is difficult to assess these 'values'. Furthermore, the emotive aspects

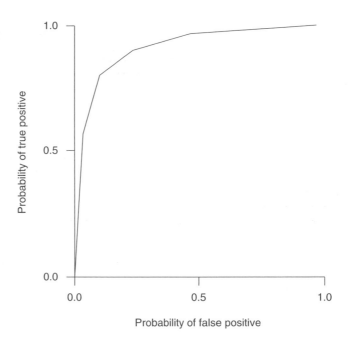

Figure 4.2 A typical receiver operating characteristic curve.

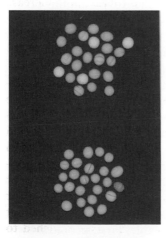

Figure 4.3 A same/different signal detection problem. The upper cluster contains four objects that are different from the others. The objects in the lower cluster are all of the same kind.

of the situation offer the prospect of regret (see below) should the decision prove incorrect.

It is worth making one further point that emerges from this model. In situations where decisions about detection have to be made on the basis of noisy data it is not possible for an observer to achieve perfect performance over a large number of observations, no matter how experienced they become. It is not uncommon to characterise individual performance using a **receiver operating characteristic** (ROC) curve, which is a plot of the rate of false positive against the rate of true positive decisions. A typical example of this is given in Figure 4.2. From this it can be seen that, while a high rate of correct decisions can be made with very low (but non-zero) false positive rates, as the correct decision rate approaches 100%, the false positive rate suddenly increases quite rapidly. Thus some wrong decisions are inevitable, and should not be taken as evidence of carelessness or lack of ability. Indeed, this is evident amongst values of acceptable performance levied by various image interpretation programmes for non-medical personnel. Prime *et al.* discovered most programmes expect between 90% and 95% accuracy agreement with the skeletal radiologist who is taken as the gold standard[3]. The methods of calculating sensitivity, specificity and accuracy, as used by programmes of study, are given in Appendix 1.

The signal detection model can be extended to cover other types of problem such as those requiring 'same/different' decisions. Figure 4.3 illustrates an example in which the task is to compare two films. In one of the films the objects are all of the same type; in the other film they may (i) also be all of the same type, or (ii) be a mixture of two different

Four

types. The two films are viewed side by side and one of the two alternatives must be chosen. Varying the exposure of the film varies the difficulty of the task.

Cognitive processes in decision making

The rational model

Early attempts[4] to formalise descriptions of decision making used the concept of the ideal decision maker as a way of describing a completely rational (i.e. unbiased) decision making process. The essential elements of this rational process are:

- list all the possible outcomes of each action open to us in the circumstances;
- estimate the probability of each outcome actually occurring;
- estimate the value (or **utility**) of each outcome – this may be negative;
- for each outcome, multiply the utility of the outcome by its probability of occurrence to get the **expected utility** of each outcome; and
- decide on the outcome with the highest expected utility.

The rational decision maker would act in such a way as to **maximise the expected utility of a decision**. However, in many cases even the most determinedly rational person would have difficulty following this procedure. In the first place we may not *know* all the possible consequences of each action. Second, we may have great difficulty in estimating the probability of each outcome occurring. Third, estimating the utility of an outcome can be very difficult. Then again, most people are *not* determinedly rational; if they were they would not do a host of things including buying lottery tickets, smoking cigarettes, having unprotected sex with strangers and climbing stepladders that are insecurely positioned (the most common cause of injury in the home in the UK).

It is not surprising that research shows people only follow the expected utility model in a limited number of closely specified cases, such as choices between gambles where the number of alternatives, their associated probabilities and their value (usually money) are fixed. When these parameters are not completely known, people have to deviate from the rational model in ways that make the problem manageable. First, people show a tendency to make decisions that satisfy their most important needs, rather than conducting an exhaustive examination of alternatives in order to optimise expected utility. Simon[5] coined the term **satisfice** to express this idea. There is plenty of evidence to demonstrate that in real life people satisfice rather than optimise when making decisions. We should remember that these needs may not always be of *direct* relevance to the problem and may, for example, include social factors such as the need to avoid losing face or the need to avoid confrontation with colleagues.

Second, people do not always value the **losses** consequent upon a wrong decision in the same way as they value the **gains** that may accrue from a correct one. Let us take as an example a simple decision with two equally probable outcomes. If outcome 1 occurs you gain £5. If outcome 2 occurs you lose £5. The expected utility of the decision is zero and according to the rational model people should be indifferent about which alternative they choose. In practice of course they are not, because what matters to them are gains and losses from a reference point, which in this case is the state of affairs before the decision. A lot of people are averse to the risk of losses and would (for example) rather pass by the chance of gaining £100 altogether, rather than risk losing £100. Thus the *perceived value* (i.e. cost) of a wrong decision can bias decision making. Kahneman and Tversky[6] developed their **prospect theory** around this phenomenon.

The asymmetry of the value function (Figure 4.4) reflects the phenomenon of **risk aversion**. This refers to the tendency of many people to

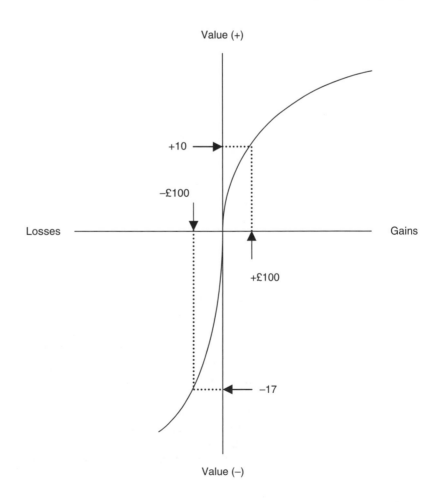

Figure 4.4 A hypothetical asymmetrical value function illustrating the prospect theory. The positive value of a gain is smaller than the negative value of the same size loss.

over-value the expected costs of losses and under-value the expected benefits of gains. It demonstrates that **psychological comfort** is important and it often makes sense for individuals to make decisions that might be theoretically sub-optimal, but which will make them happier given their psychological needs. An example may be the apparent hedging of decisions by using statements that suggest a certain injury pattern or erring on the side of caution to say that the balance of features raises the index of suspicion. This would allow one to reiterate the description such that a decision is taken that has no overall detrimental effect on patient management.

Estimating probability

The other major issue in decision making has to do with the way in which we estimate probabilities. In some cases we can define the probability of something happening in an objective way: picking the winning sequence of numbers in the National Lottery is one obvious example. The probability of this happening is 1 divided by the number of ways you can pick six numbers out of 49. In other words it is the number of target outcomes (1) divided by the number of possible outcomes (13 983 816). To be precise, this statement assumes that the numbers are picked at random, i.e. each possible sequence of six numbers is as likely to occur as any other. There are very few situations where this kind of procedure is practical because it depends on one being able to specify the complete list of possible outcomes and being able to say that each one is equally probable, by virtue of the way the draw is made. In other cases we can estimate the probability of something (say, the occurrence of a disease) by making a careful study of a sample of people from some population and discovering the proportion of them that have the disease. The *prevalence* of a disease is thus an estimate of the probability that a person drawn at random from that population will have that disease. Counting cases as they occur is a cruder version of the same procedure, which yields a progressively more accurate estimate as more data are collected.

Conditional probability and Bayes' theorem

Patients are not 'people drawn at random', however. They are patients because they have signs and symptoms of illness and, at least in theory, the information gained from tests and examinations can be used to increase the probability of a correct diagnosis. If we can estimate the probabilities associated with the outcome of tests then we can combine them using Bayes' theorem which provides a way of working with what are known as **conditional** probabilities. It is useful in circumstances where we know the probability of two events occurring independently, but need to know the probability of one event occurring *given that* we know that the other event already has. This kind of situation frequently occurs where tests are used to diagnose disease states, and the clinician has to decide whether a positive test indicates the presence of disease. Of course Bayes' theorem is a statistical tool and as such it describes how people *should* act rather than how they actually do. An appreciation of the distinction can be very instructive. Bayes' theorem is usually expressed by this equation:

$$p(A/B) = \frac{p(B/A) \times p(A)}{p(B)}$$

An example devised by Kahneman and Tversky in 1974[6] illustrates how the theorem may be applied in practice. In a small town there are two taxi firms, the Green Cab Company (who have 85% of the taxis) and the Blue Cab Company (who have 15% of the taxis.) One night there is a hit-and-run accident involving a taxi, and a single eyewitness says that the cab was a blue one. The question is: What is the probability that the taxi involved in the accident was a blue one?

If we did not have the eyewitness we could only say that the probability of the taxi being blue is 0.15, because that is the proportion of blue taxis in the town. The eyewitness gives us additional information but, remembering that eyewitness testimony is often unreliable and that the accident took place at night, we arrange to test the eyewitness. The outcome is that the witness succeeds in correctly identifying the two colours 80% of the time and fails to do so 20% of the time. Looking back at the equation let us say that A is the event that the cab *is* blue and B is the event that the witness *says* that the cab is blue. We know that the probability of the cab being blue is:

$$p(A) = 0.15$$

and that the probability of the witness saying the cab is blue, given that it actually *is* blue, is:

$$p(B|A) = 0.80$$

What we want to know is $p(A|B)$, that is, the probability that the cab is blue *given that the witness says it is*.

To calculate this we need one further probability $p(B)$, which is the probability that the witness will say the cab was blue. This is calculated by adding together the probability that witness says the cab was blue when it was blue and the probability that the witness says the cab was blue when it was actually green:

$$p(B) = (0.15 \times 0.80) + (0.85 \times 0.20) = 0.29$$

Now we can write:

$$p(A/B) = \frac{0.80 \times 0.15}{0.29} = 0.41$$

So despite what the witness says, the final outcome is that the taxi was more likely to be green than blue. People generally find this result surprising, partly because they are inclined to believe eyewitnesses anyway, and also because they are unable to use the information about eyewitness reliability in a quantitative way and simply resort to the judgement that '80% is pretty accurate'.

The disparity between intuitive judgement and the result of a Bayesian calculation can be very important. We can easily apply the logic of the taxi example to a clinical situation that is concerned with the question 'What is the probability that a woman has breast cancer, given a positive test?'[7].

$p(A)$ is the probability that a woman without symptoms has breast cancer, and national statistics indicate that this is about 0.01. $p(B|A)$ is the **specificity** of the test, that is, the probability that the patient has cancer given a positive test. Let us say this is 0.9. Finally we need to know $p(B)$, the probability of a positive test from a mammogram. Following the same reasoning used in the taxi example, this is calculated as the sum of the probabilities of a true positive test and a false positive test. The probability of a true positive test is the sensitivity of the test multiplied by the probability of having breast cancer. That is, $0.90 \times 0.01 = 0.009$. The probability of a false positive test is (1 − specificity of the test) multiplied by the probability of *not* having breast cancer – that is, $(1 − 0.9) \times 0.99 = 0.099$. The sum of these two probabilities gives the probability of getting a positive result from a mammogram, which equals 0.108. We can then apply Bayes' theorem to find the probability of a patient having breast cancer given a *positive* mammogram:

$$\frac{0.01 \times 0.9}{0.108} = 0.08$$

Again, people often find the result of this calculation very surprising particularly in the light of the emphasis often given to screening programmes.

Heuristics and biases

In many cases, however, we have no firm data and we simply have to estimate probabilities as best we can. One way in which we do this is by using rules of thumb called **heuristics**[8]. Heuristics reduce the time needed to make reasonably accurate decisions, and they generally yield quite good estimates. However, they are also prone to very predictable biases.

Representativeness heuristic

The first of these rules of thumb is called the **representativeness** heuristic. This involves people judging probabilities by the degree to which A resembles B. So if A is a person and B is a group then the decision might

---

Box 4.1   Representativeness heuristic.

John is 45 years old and a professor at an American university. He is small of stature and quite shy. He writes poetry. Which of the following is more likely to be true?

- John is of Chinese descent.
- John teaches English Literature and is of Chinese descent.

---

be whether person A is a member of group B. The example in Box 4.1 provides an illustration of how the representativeness heuristic can allow biases to creep into decision making.

Ninety per cent of people who were given this question ticked the second box even though this breaks one of the fundamental rules of probability theory: the co-occurrence of two events cannot be more likely than the probability of either event alone. This phenomenon (called the conjunction fallacy) has been demonstrated in a wide range of situations and we should be aware, as Tversky and Kahneman[8] point out, that as the amount of detail in a scenario increases, its probability steadily decreases. However, its representativeness (i.e. how we imagine the event) increases with increasing detail, and therefore so does its *apparent* likelihood.

Reliance on representativeness may, amongst other things, lead to people ignoring base rates when making decisions. So, for example, if faced with a description of symptoms which seems equally representative of two possible illnesses there is a strong tendency for clinicians to judge that the patient could equally well have one illness or the other without taking into account the fact that one illness may be more common than the other. This tendency will introduce bigger biases when base rates are very high or very low.

Availability heuristic

The second rule of thumb is called the **availability** heuristic. This involves people judging the probability of an event by the ease with which they can recall instances of it happening. On the whole this strategy works quite effectively, with instances of common events being easier to recall than instances of uncommon ones. However, there are other reasons why we might readily recall an event and these reasons can bias our judgement. For example, events that occurred recently are more readily recalled than those that happened longer ago, and so things which we have come across recently (for example, a particular illness) will tend to be judged as more frequent (and hence more probable) than things we have not experienced recently – or even at all.

Events which grab the headlines in the papers are 'more available' than those which do not, and are likely to be judged as more probable. For example, shark attacks are highly publicised and are more easy to

Four

Four

imagine than being killed by a falling aeroplane part, yet in the USA the chances of dying from the latter are 30 times higher than the former. Researchers in a large American hospital asked surgeons to estimate the mortality rate for the hospital's surgical service as a whole. Surgeons from high mortality specialities such as cardiovascular surgery and neurosurgery estimated the overall rate to be double that estimated by those in low mortality areas such as orthopaedics and urology[9]. One might expect that a surgeon's own experiences would be more available than the experiences of others, and in this case they seemed to exert a biasing influence over their judgement.

Regret and the omission bias

We often review the outcome of our decisions in order to improve our future performance. Unfortunately some of our decisions may have unforeseen negative consequences, and we may go over what we might have done differently to see whether we missed some crucial factor, or whether our evaluation of the evidence was in some other way faulty. This activity is known as **counterfactual thinking**, and if we *can* imagine a way in which we could have acted differently and avoided the negative consequences then we attribute the consequences to our own failure, and experience **regret**. The anticipation of regret can introduce another kind of bias into decision making. It seems that people have a tendency to control their actions so as to minimise potential regret and when framing a decision, they focus on the consequences of actions taken to the exclusion of actions not taken. There are several possible reasons for this. People may feel more personally responsible (because of a perceived causal link) for the consequences of things that they do than for things they do not do. And society tends to hold people more accountable for their actions than for their failure to act. It may also be more difficult to imagine bad outcomes as a result of inaction than as a result of action. However, the overall result is known as **omission bias**, that is, a tendency not to act in order to minimise the regret felt should an action lead to a negative outcome. For example, parents may be reluctant to vaccinate their children if they feel there is a small probability of an adverse reaction even when the probability of a bad outcome is much higher if the vaccine is withheld. One consequence of this bias is that, in retrospect, people tend to recollect more regret as the result of inaction than of action.

Confirmatory bias

Confirmatory bias refers to a type of selective thinking whereby people tend to search out and pay attention to information that confirms their beliefs and to ignore, not look for or under-value the relevance of anything that contradicts those beliefs. It also entails ignoring the nonoccurrence of events, which are more easily forgotten than occurrences. The confirmation bias typically occurs because we have difficulty in dealing with negative information (i.e. information that does not confirm our hypothesis) and because we tend to be poor at extracting diagnostic value out of the absence of information. Typically, the absence of information is thought to signal that we need to look for more data, rather than treating such absences as valuable pieces of information that will help inform a decision.

Confirmatory bias can lead to errors in reading images for two reasons. First, it may lead the practitioner to 'shut down' on the scan of an image as soon as a piece of evidence is found which indicates a plausible diagnosis. The second reason is linked to the question of how much clinical information should be available before the image is examined. Clinical information may establish expectations about what may be discovered in the image and as a result the practitioner may be biased towards discovering data that confirm those expectations.

Social processes in decision making

Group polarisation and the risky shift

Group decision making differs from individual decision making and, in general, decisions made by groups are more extreme than those that would be made by the individual members of the group acting in isolation. This phenomenon was originally known as the **risky shift** because studies of choices involving risk showed that group decisions were more risky than the individual decisions of group members. However, it is now known that the effect is a more general one and that if the members of the group are inclined to caution then the group decision will be more cautious still. Thus the effect of group discussion is to amplify the original feelings of participants, and for this reason it is now known as **group polarisation.**

Although group polarisation is a well-established occurrence, there is no single established reason for it. This is perhaps because of the variety of ways in which people choose to behave when they know that others are watching (and perhaps evaluating) them. For example, people generally need to compare their opinions with those of others and to be perceived positively by them. Consequently they may be motivated to *change* their stance to fit in with what they perceive to be the most socially desirable position within the group. The overall group position may become polarised because of the combined effect of these comparisons and the effect may be increased when the group has members of differing status. There is some support for this from research, which shows that merely *knowing* the opinions of others (without having heard their arguments) can produce the polarisation effect.

Four

In some cases polarisation may come about as a result of the persuasiveness of the arguments which are put forward during the discussions. In general, arguments will support the views already held by group members. To the extent that these arguments support the view you already hold, they will strengthen your own position. People may also produce arguments you had not thought of before which may make your position more extreme. This explanation is, then, that the arguments themselves, rather than the individual positions, give rise to polarisation.

Groupthink

Group decision making does not, however, always produce polarisation. In some cases a group may produce unrealistic decisions by failing to consider information or arguments that do not fit in with the group's initial view. Among the symptoms of groupthink are:

- An illusion of unanimity, where silence is seen as consent.
- Collective efforts to rationalise warnings that things might be going wrong.
- A shared illusion of the group's superior expertise, leading to over-optimism and excessive risk taking.
- Stereotyping of any opponents in negative terms, e.g. as uninformed or stupid.
- The existence of self-appointed 'mindguards' who protect the group from undesirable information.
- An unquestioned belief that the group is acting for the overall good of all concerned.

Groupthink is most likely to occur when the group is cohesive, has a strong leadership and cuts itself off from outside influence.

Janis[10] coined the term 'groupthink' in his analysis of serious errors made by the US administration in the 1970s, but it would be a mistake to believe that the phenomenon is confined to high status groups making decisions of grave importance. Examples of groupthink have been found in a number of clinical decision making groups[11]. One of the effects of groupthink in this context is to engender a culture in which no one challenges anyone else's clinical decisions, this being presented to the outside world as a reflection of the mutual respect in which group members hold each other. In fact, group members may fear the consequences of going against the norms of thinking and behaving, even if the group's work deteriorates to the point of dysfunction.

A number of preventive measures can safeguard against groupthink. The first is to encourage dissent and criticism. The second is that group leaders should refrain from stating their personal preferences at the outset in discussions. In some Japanese companies, for example, group members express opinions in ascending order of rank so that no one censors their own opinion for fear of disagreeing with someone higher up in the company. Third, group members should periodically discuss the group's deliberations with other colleagues and report the results of this (a form of peer review) back to the group. Each of these measures legitimises disagreement and capitalises on the fact that dissent reduces conformity.

Concluding remarks

The theme of this chapter is simple. When making decisions in a professional capacity we need to set aside the habits of everyday life – no matter how well they serve us – and reflect on what we are doing. All judgements, even those made at the most basic sensory level, are vulnerable to bias due to individual and social factors: there is no such thing as a dispassionate human decision maker. Computer-based medical decision making tools may help evaluate evidence in a way that is independent of individual preferences, but they are no substitute for the need to be aware of one's own values and how they affect the way one makes decisions in difficult cases. Furthermore, while perfection may be a worthy goal, some types of decision (e.g. X-ray screening) must be made even though there may simply not be enough information in the image. In such cases a small proportion of mistakes is inevitable and one should not set unrealistic targets for oneself or others.

Cognitive biases can be reduced, if not completely eliminated, by taking steps to ensure that evidence is collected and evaluated in the most systematic way possible. Two key principles to keep in mind are the importance of looking for disconfirming evidence and paying close attention to base rates.

Making decisions in small groups has its benefits, the most obvious being that one person may find evidence that another has missed or produce arguments that others have not thought of. But there are potential costs in the form of judgements that go beyond the evidence because the participants are too sure of their own positions, too scared of losing face to disagree with a superior or too entrenched in a culture of self-serving consensus to consider all the alternatives. The best safeguard against such dangers is simple rules of deliberation, that encourage rather than suppress dissent, to which everyone subscribes.

Editor's note

Decision making, by its very nature, is a concept that is difficult to understand, being subject to many individual vagaries as outlined in this chapter. Some of these inconsistencies are being negotiated by the adoption of the double reporting approach, particularly in the mammographic and gastro-intestinal fields. Indeed, some imaging departments operate long-term auditing procedures on the performance of their non-medically

Four

trained reporting staff in such a way as to create a double reporting methodology to service provision. However, the discussion surrounding the position of social standing within the double reporting team does suggest that it would be possible for members of that team to be over-ridden in the decision making process. If this occurs then where does this effectively leave the team with respect to the service it provides other than taking more manpower to do the same job? There must, therefore, be acceptance by all with respect to how each individual contributes to that team as indicated in the concluding comments of this chapter.

References

1   Hunink, M.G., Glasziou, P.P., Siegel, J.E., Weeks, J.C., Pliskin, J.S., Elstein, A.S. and Weinstein, M.C. (2001) *Decision Making in Health and Medicine*. Cambridge University Press, Cambridge.

2   Shafir, E. (1994) Reason-based choice. In: Johnson-Laird, P.N. and Shafir, E. (eds.) *Reasoning and Decision Making*. Blackwell Publishers, Oxford.

3   Prime, N.J., Paterson, A.M. and Henderson, P.I. (1999) The development of a curriculum – a case study of six centres providing courses in radiographic reporting. *Radiography London* 5(2), 63–70.

4   von Neumann, J. and Morgenstern, O. (1949) *The Theory of Games and Economic Behavior*. Princeton University Press, Princeton.

5   Simon, H.A. (1956) Rational choice and the structure of the environment. *Psychological Review* 63, 129–38.

6   Kahneman, D. and Tversky, A. (1979) Prospect theory: an analysis of decision under risk. *Econometrica* 47, 263–91.

7   Everitt, B.S. (1999) *Chance Rules: An Informal Guide to Probability, Risk and Statistics*. Copernicus, New York.

8   Tversky, A. and Kahneman, D. (1974) Judgement under uncertainty: heuristics and biases. *Science* 185, 1124–30.

9   Detmer, D.E., Fryback, D.G. and Gassner, K. (1978) Heuristics and biases in medical decision making. *Journal of Medical Education* 53, 682–3.

10   Janis, I. L. (1982) *Groupthink: Analysis of Policy Decisions and Fiascoes*, 2nd edn. Houghton Mifflin, Boston.

11   Griffiths, J. and Luker, K. (1994) Intra-professional research in district nursing: in whose interests? *Journal of Advanced Nursing* 20(b), 1038–45.

5 Pattern Recognition

Dr Ian Christensen

Introduction

The term **pattern** implies 'organisation'. The human visual system is very good at recognising patterns, that is, determining when elements in the visual field are related to each other and are therefore likely to be components of the same object. Some of this ability is a function of the way in which the visual system is constructed, but in large part our abilities, while obviously underpinned by the structure of the system, are learnt. This makes sense from a biological perspective since it enables humans to adapt, from birth, to the particular environment in which they will have to function.

Figure 5.1 provides an illustration of what we mean by visual organisation. Most people identify this picture as being of a dog in an open space, with a small tree on the left. If you look closely at the **elements** of the picture you can see that there are very few dog-like components present; much of what is there consists of small, unconnected black blobs. However, our experience of small animals and our general surroundings enables us to construct an interpretation of the visual field that is consistent with the evidence. Pattern recognition and object identification is thus an active process concerned with what has been termed **effort after meaning**.

Figure 5.2 provides another example; this contains much less information and is consequently far harder to identify. (If the reader can make no sense of it, the solution is given at the end of the chapter.) Figure 5.3 contains no information at all about the likely relation of the elements and consequently the visual system 'trys out' alternative schemes of organisation. None of these are stable, however.

In addition to our ability to make sense out of ambiguous or poorly defined stimuli, our ability to recognise objects is extremely versatile. We can identify objects in various orientations, when they are poorly lit or partly obscured by other objects. Suppose you go to visit someone at their office which you have never seen before. As you arrive they are just

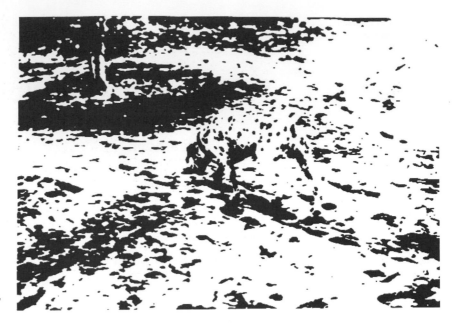

Figure 5.1   An example of perceptual problem solving. (Photograph by Ronald James, cited from Gleitman, 1999.)

Five

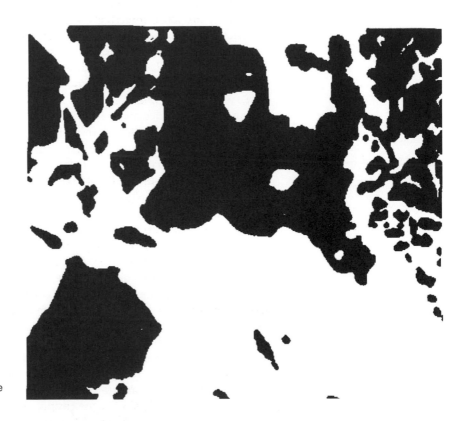

Figure 5.2   A second example of a perceptual problem.

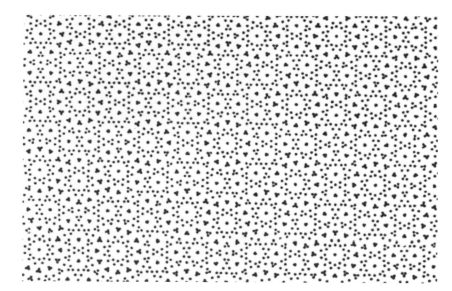

Figure 5.3 A third example of a perceptual problem. There are a number of equally plausible ways of organising the elements of this figure and the visual system alternates between them.

leaving on a brief errand and invite you to go inside and sit down for a few moments to wait. None of us would have any problem identifying what is a chair, even though the room, and the furniture, are unfamiliar. We take this ability for granted, but the task involves an analysis of the visual field and the identification, using memory, of the objects most likely to be chairs. Unless the furniture is of the most avant-garde design we are unlikely to make a mistake. Our visual system operates in a very flexible way, and accounting for this flexibility is a central issue for visual theory.

The neural basis of pattern recognition

The process of pattern recognition begins with the retina and the neural connections that link its light-sensitive elements (the rods and cones) together. Figure 5.4 is a simplified diagram of the retina showing the principal components. Light, shown as entering from the left of the diagram, passes through layers of neurones of four distinct types before arriving at the light-sensitive cells themselves. These intermediate neurones provide a rich system of interconnectivity so that the outputs from adjacent cells in the retina may interact. The activity of a single ganglion cell may represent the combined activity of a large number of rods and cones, and so a single ganglion cell may respond to light that is incident upon a relatively large area of the retina; this area is called the **receptive field** of the cell. Furthermore, the output of these cells feeds into cells in area V1 of the visual cortex in a hierarchical fashion, leading to the terms **simple**, **complex** and **hypercomplex** for successively more specialised cells

Five

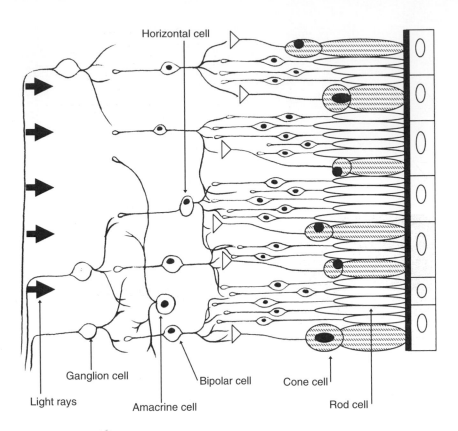

Figure 5.4   A schematic diagram of the retina.[5]

that respond to increasingly more specific combinations of features in their receptive fields (Figure 5.5) In effect the visual system performs a type of **feature analysis** on its input.

Receptive fields may react with a burst of activity following the onset of a stimulus (an ON response) or following the termination of a stimulus (an OFF response). The typical receptive field has a roughly circular centre in which the stimulus onset causes an ON response. The outer part of the field gives the opposite result, that is, the onset does not produce a response, but the offset does. Some receptive fields have the opposite organisation (Figure 5.6). The complex interconnectivity within the visual pathway means that a ganglion cell does not have exclusive rights to the output of a group of receptors, and a particular receptor can contribute to the receptive field of several ganglion cells.

These interactions within areas of receptive fields serve, amongst other things, to emphasise the contours within an image. The neural mechanism that achieves this is termed **lateral inhibition**. Cells responding at, for instance, the boundary between areas of light and dark in the visual image will *inhibit* the output of adjacent cells, effectively sharpening the boundary by suppressing stray weak signals in its immediate vicinity. For example, when we perceive contrast between two shades of grey, we experience anomalies that are due to lateral inhibition. The two inner

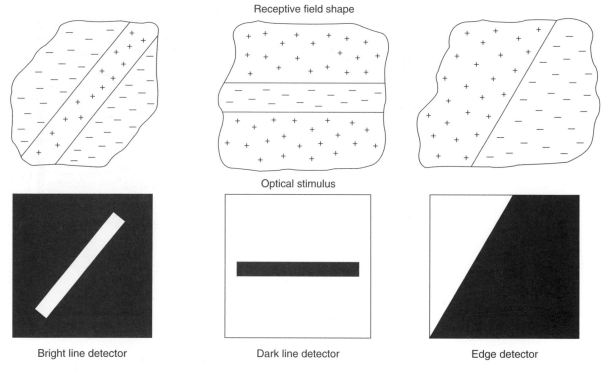

Figure 5.5   Sample receptive fields of 'simple' cortical cells.

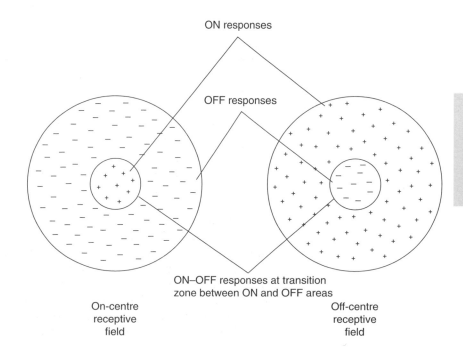

Figure 5.6   Two types of centre-surround visual fields.

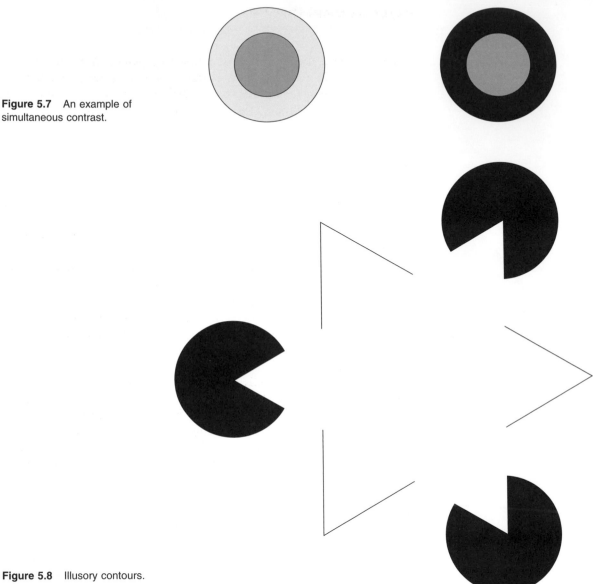

Figure 5.7 An example of simultaneous contrast.

Figure 5.8 Illusory contours. (After Kanizsa, 1976.)

Five

circles in Figure 5.7 are the same, but there is a tendency to see the one on the left as darker than the one on the right. The existence of illusory contours (Figure 5.8) provides a striking example in which not only do we experience shapes when the contours that define them are almost entirely absent but we also experience contrast differences between these shapes and the background when they are both quite clearly of the same shade of white. For a more detailed and highly readable account of the structure of the visual pathway and the visual cortex the reader might like to consult Coren *et al.*[2]

Psychological theories

Given that the structure of the visual system provides, *de facto*, a feature analysis of the incoming pattern of light, the interesting question arises as to whether what we perceive is somehow built up from these elementary units or whether the natural units of perception are forms themselves.

Distinctive features

If we consider shapes as regions of the image on the retina that are bounded by contours then these shapes have properties of spatial extent, texture, colour and so on. We can refer to these properties as **features** and they enable us to discriminate objects from each other. In some cases discrimination requires a small number of features (discriminating between a chair and a filing cabinet, for example) and sometimes it requires rather more. Research suggests that only a relatively small number of fundamental features are needed to perform most discrimination tasks; these include colour, brightness, orientation, length, curvature, line endings, intersections and line closures.[3] This might seem an appealing approach if these features can be traced back to their source in the receptive fields of cells in the visual pathway. This type of processing, which registers the presence of features and patterns in the sensory input, is termed **data-driven** (or **bottom-up**) because the incoming information is processed according to rules that are determined by the structure of the sensory pathway. We should remember, however, that there is an important difference between neural feature detectors and the hypothetical detectors assumed by this model, and that is that the responses of neural feature detectors are *not* independent of other features in the stimulus, while in the psychological model they are.

Identifying objects might certainly begin with analysis of features in this fashion. However, there are a number of reasons why this type of analysis on its own cannot be entirely responsible for our ability to recognise patterns and hence identify objects. The most important of these is the fact that we are clearly able to make use of our past experiences and our knowledge of the world we live in when interpreting visual inputs. These **concept-driven** (or **top-down**) processes are responsible for integrating features into perceptual objects, often in conjunction with expectations about what is probable in a given context. Context is a very important factor in the identification process, especially when the image is ambiguous or only seen briefly (see Figure 5.1 again, and also Figure 5.9). Furthermore, it is clear that when we need to *search* for objects in the visual field we have at least some choice about which features to use in the task. In Figure 5.10 the target is a white letter D: consider what features are needed to identify the letter in each block.

Five

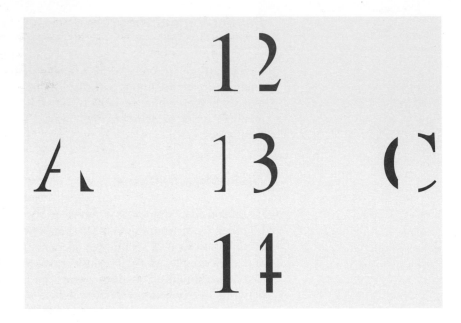

Figure 5.9   The perception of the central item depends on whether it is seen in the horizontal or vertical context.

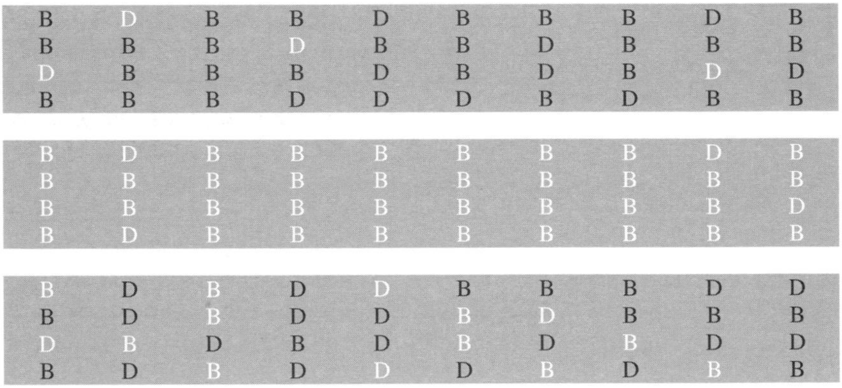

Figure 5.10   The top block requires searching for brightness only, the middle block requires searching for shape only. The bottom block requires searching for the conjunction of both features. There are four targets in each block.

Five

Gestalt theory

The distinctive features approach emerged from the analysis of the relatively simple task of recognising letters. Natural shapes are much more complex, and the issue of the relation between features becomes important. One influential view of this problem became known as **Gestalt** theory, which was based on the premise that the visual array will always be perceived in terms of the most simple and stable patterns. From this theory emerged the **principles of perceptual organisation**, which describe how we respond to the relation *between* the elements of the perceptual field rather than to the elements themselves. The most important of these principles are (with reference to Figure 5.11):

- The **principle of proximity** (Figure 5.11a–c): elements that are close together are more likely to be seen as belonging together. In

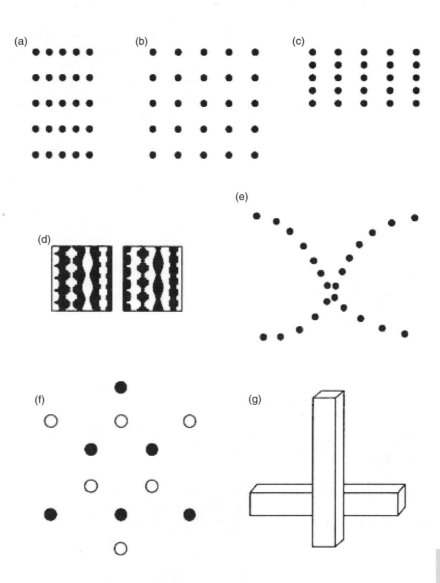

Figure 5.11(a–f) Examples of the Gestalt principles of perceptual organisation.

Figure 5.11a we see rows of dots because the horizontal spacing is narrower than the vertical spacing. In Figure 5.11c we see columns of dots because the vertical spacing is narrower. In Figure 5.11b the organisation disappears because the horizontal and vertical spacings are equal.

- The **principle of symmetry** (Figure 5.11d): elements that form symmetrical units are more likely to be seen as belonging together than those which do not. In the left panel of the figure we readily see white bars against a black background, but it is almost impossible to see black bars against a white background for more than a few seconds. In the right panel the opposite is true, demonstrating that the stable pattern is determined by symmetry rather than colour.

Five

- The **principle of good continuation** (Figure 5.11e): elements appear grouped together to form smooth and uninterrupted lines whenever possible. In this example it is easiest to see two curved lines that cross. Although other interpretations are possible they are not easily perceived.
- The **principle of similarity** (Figure 5.11f): elements that are similar are more likely to be seen as part of the same figure. In this illustration we are more likely to see two triangles (one made up of black dots and one made up of white dots) than a six-pointed star.
- The **principle of closure** (Figure 5.11g): elements group together in a way that favours the more complete (or 'closed') figure. In this example there are three rectangular shapes but the principles of continuation and closure favour the perception of a horizontal bar lying *behind* the vertical one.

The pattern in Figure 5.3 also demonstrates these principles in action. The Gestalt theorists emphasised that it was the relation *between* the elements in the visual field that defined the form that we perceive, declaring that the whole is greater than the sum of its parts. They used the demonstration of ambiguous figures (Figure 5.12) to illustrate that one visual stimulus could give rise to more than one distinct perception and that, therefore, the thing that we perceived could not be determined (at least not entirely) by its individual elements.

Five

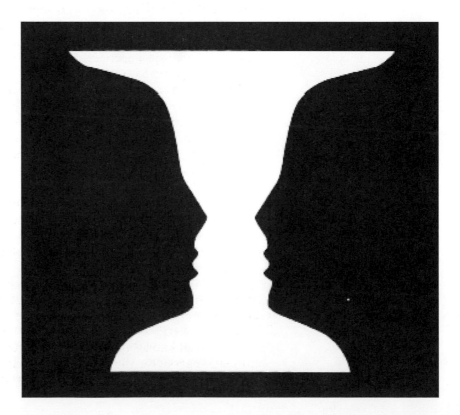

Figure 5.12 An ambiguous figure that alternates between two faces seen in profile and a vase. It is not possible to maintain a stable perception of one alternative for more than a few seconds at a time.

There is no doubt that the Gestalt psychologists produced some powerful demonstrations to illustrate that there are some processes involved in pattern recognition that are **automatic** and which can only be over-ridden with difficulty, if at all. However, most of the pattern recognition that concerns us in everyday as well as professional life is concerned with visual analyses that are based on experience and therefore have a substantial learnt component. While it is true that these analyses will be underpinned by the basic processes carried out by the complex connections in the visual pathway, and may be further mediated by the Gestalt principles mentioned above, nevertheless it is still true that in many respects we have to learn to see.

The template model

Another view of the nature of the top-down processes that are responsible for integrating features is known as the **template** theory. This assumes that once we have seen something, we store in our memory a miniature representation, or template, of the features of that object. This template does not, of course, resemble a photograph, but the spatial arrangement of the various parts of the visual stimulus is assumed to be preserved. These stored representations are given labels that derive from the observer's personal experience. When we see that object again we recognise it by matching the visual input with likely templates, finally choosing the one that provides the best fit with the visual data. The final act of recognition is characterised as a decision making process because it may be based on imperfect or incomplete information and, accordingly, can be prone to error.

Although this seems an intuitively reasonable idea, there is a difficulty. We can recognise a very great number of patterns under a wide variety of situations (lighting, distance, angle of view, and so on) and the basic template theory only deals with this by proposing an indefinitely large number of templates. The memory capacity of the brain is finite and probably does not have the capacity to store all the templates that would be needed for us to recognise vast numbers of patterns in a huge variety of orientations. Furthermore, the more templates you acquire, the longer it should take to recognise any particular pattern because there are more alternatives templates to consider. This does not appear to happen, and it is generally agreed that the multiple template idea is probably not true.

A possible variation on the basic template idea is that each pattern is represented by a single stored template, but that the visual image is in some way normalised (e.g. rotated and scaled to a standard orientation and size) before the matching process takes place. This certainly reduces the memory requirement, but instead will require a great deal of computation. In addition the normalisation process would need to have some information about the stimulus *before* it could rearrange the internal representation. In other words, some form of identification would already had to have taken place.

Five

A ᴀ ᴀ A **ᴬ** ᴀ **ᴀ** A A
A ᴀ ᴀ ᴀ ᴀ ᴀ **ᴀ** **A** A

Figure 5.13 Upper and lower case examples of the letter 'A' in a variety of fonts.

The prototype model

Template theory treats each stimulus as a separate case, regardless of any features that it may have in common with other stimuli. Thus each of the characters in Figure 5.13 would have its *own* template and the recognition of each stimulus would be independent of all the others. It is this separate and independent treatment of each stimulus which gives rise to the huge memory demands of the template model.

The prototype model, on the other hand, starts from the position that the similarities among related stimuli are essential for pattern recognition. If all stimuli are regarded as members of classes of stimuli, then any single stimulus will reflect (to a greater or lesser extent) the **shared attributes** of the class. The **prototype** is a reflection of the modal values of the shared attributes of the class. Classes of stimuli are defined by rules of membership termed **schemata** and pattern recognition, according to the prototype model, is not only a process of *ex*tracting information but also of *ab*stracting information. Pattern recognition depends on a process of abstracting the essential characteristics of stimuli and formulating the rules (schemata) that characterise classes of stimuli with low **variability** between stimuli within the class and high variability between classes.

On the face of things the prototype model is the more plausible because it only requires us to store the much less numerous prototypes, together with their schemata, instead of a great number of templates. There is also experimental evidence that we do form prototypes when faced with brand new patterns. The general form of the experiments is as follows. First, two simple but different patterns are devised: these are the prototypes. Then additional patterns are formulated that are **distortions** of these two prototypes. Half of the distorted patterns are set aside and the others are mixed up and shown to observers one by one. They are asked to say whether each pattern represents prototype one or prototype two – neither of which they have seen. Naturally they can only guess at first, but they are told whether they are right or wrong after each presentation and after several repeated presentations they learn to classify each pattern correctly. At this point observers are asked to classify some of the patterns they have already seen, some of the patterns that were set aside from the beginning and the prototype patterns themselves. What happens is that observers classify the old patterns and the prototypes correctly, but are much less accurate with the new patterns. This suggests that in learning to classify the original patterns (the variations on the prototype) they also learnt the prototypes themselves. In other words an observer will form a prototype when presented with a recognition problem involving members of a class of related stimuli, because it helps them with the problem – not because they have been asked to do so. Further research has shown that when patterns are generated from a prototype by introducing several successive distortions then correct classification rates for stimuli with the same number of distortions are similar whether or not they have been seen before. Thus the prototype is used to classify and identify new patterns[4].

Computational models

The computational approach to the problem of pattern recognition and the perception of form starts with a set of questions about the kind of information processing a perceptual system must carry out in order to accomplish the task. The problems are addressed in terms of the way in which a computer might process such information and this requires formal, precise and unambiguous specification of both the information and the computational process.

The most influential theorist in this field has been David Marr[5] who suggested that descriptions of perceptual processing must be addressed at three levels: the computational theory, representations and algorithms, and hardware implementation. At the first level we are concerned with specifying what is to be recognised, the information that may be available in the retinal image and the information needed to achieve the correct solution. At the second level we have to examine the ways in which information can be represented in the system and the kinds of calculations that must be accomplished to achieve the solution. And at the third level we must consider the specification of the device that will implement the solution. This approach has of course been heavily influenced by computer scientists and engineers whose goal is to develop machines that can 'see'. These attempts have been successful in a range of industrial settings, and are beginning to influence the ways in which medical imaging programs are written. Their contribution to psychological knowledge will ultimately be judged on whether or not they provide us with insights into how the brain actually processes visual information.

Concluding remarks

The reader will have gathered that pattern recognition is one of those areas of psychology where there are a number of competing theories, but no definitive answers. The simple act of recognising this object as a book can be described in a number of ways, each deriving from a different theoretical perspective and each with points to recommend it. The overall difficulty lies with the issue of generality: different approaches are useful when describing some observations but not others. However, we should not let this lack of a complete theory of pattern perception deter us from making use of what we do know.

In the first place we should be aware that there are some perceptual processes (both sensory and cognitive) that operate to help us make sense of incomplete visual data. These processes fill in missing data, sharpen up fuzzy edges, create links between different elements of the visual field and generally encourage us to generate (and believe in) perceptions that are, on the **balance of probability**, representations of the external world.

Five

Figure 5.2 (p. 48) provides an example of this. Most people see in this figure the head of a heavily bearded man; this is easier to perceive when the picture is in a small format, as opposed to when projected in a lecture theatre. In the latter circumstance some people can never see the head even when the outline is traced on the screen and the various features pointed out. It has proved difficult to trace the provenance of this picture, and one source suggests it is actually of melting snow in the Alps, as viewed from the window of an aeroplane. Whatever the truth of that, the fact remains that some people 'see' the man and some do not and this cannot be dismissed by suggesting that the latter have perceptual processes that are in some way deficient. We must simply accept that there can be individual differences in the perception of ambiguous visual stimuli. In the specific domain of interpreting medical images, this knowledge cannot be ignored and it should alert us to the need for well-structured (and non-judgemental) monitoring systems that can detect anomalies in reporting.

Second, our perceptual processes are designed to help us make sense of our environment and sometime they mislead us. The ultrasound scan in Figure 5.14 illustrates this. An ambiguous object is suspended in a vessel of water. The lines that form the edges of the object are incomplete in some places, but it is difficult to avoid the conclusion that the object is a cube.

In fact, the object is only two-dimensional (Figure 5.15) and contains no perspective cues to support the interpretation of a three-dimensional figure. A 'cube' is simply the most likely explanation of the evidence and unless this explanation is carefully and consciously considered the evidence may be misconstrued.

Five

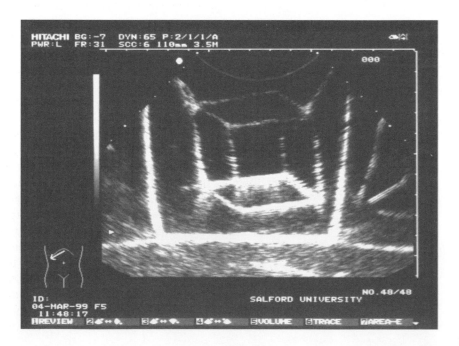

Figure 5.14 Our perceptual processes help to make sense of ambiguous images such as this ultrasound of an object suspended in a vessel of water.

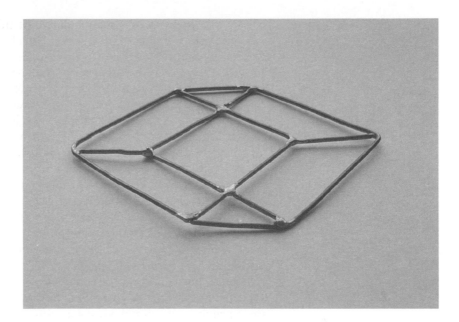

Figure 5.15 The object in Figure 5.14.

Third, research supports the idea that prototypes are an important part of pattern identification and object recognition. As we have seen, prototypes are mental abstractions that embody the essential qualities of a category, and for any given individual a prototype defines a norm for that category of object by specifying what attributes a category member should possess, and the degree to which it should possess them. However, we must not lose sight of the fact that prototypes emerge from a person's experience and for an individual to form a prototype that is *representative* of a class of objects in the external world, it follows that they must have experience that is also representative. As children grow up it is easy to observe examples of developing schemata. Naming animals provides a good demonstration. With just a little experience children are able to form a prototype called 'dog' that enables them to distinguish reliably between dogs and other small animals. But they need much more experience to form prototypes of different breeds of dog. Some of this experience may come from seeing lots of dogs, but generally the process would also involve the short-cut of being taught by someone who knows. Training can be used to facilitate the formation of prototypes by organising the experience of the student and producing exemplars that the student would not normally encounter. Well-structured training is particularly valuable for establishing what is *normal*. In professional situations that tend to focus on disease, it is easy to forget that we need a reliable prototype of what is normal in order to help us judge what is not. In order to form such prototypes we need to experience a good deal of what is normal for that class of objects and rather than simply wait for them to come along, we arrange for them to be available for study.

Five

This brings us finally to the interesting question of whether we can facilitate the formation of prototypes by having someone tell us the rules (schemata) that define them. In traditional teaching this might take the form of a lecturer saying 'X belongs to class Y if and only if it has these properties, within these limits', giving a few examples and then referring the student to a textbook. What we know about prototype formation would strongly argue against this approach, which attempts to by-pass the natural mechanism rather than work with it. Prototype formation is an active process and the student must participate in that process rather than simply observing someone else talking about it. It follows therefore that effectively structured teaching will present the student with materials that have been selected as good examples of the prototype in terms of both the essential features and the range of possible variation. Theory suggests that establishing a stable prototype is an important precursor for learning to discriminate between examples that do and do not belong to a particular class, such as normal or diseased tissue. Even though the recognition of disease and other abnormalities is one of the principal reasons for producing medical images, placing an emphasis on the recognition of pathological states at the expense of establishing the normal prototype may be counterproductive as an educational strategy.

References

1   Hubel, D.H. and Weisel, T.N. (1962) Receptive fields, binocular interaction and functional architecture in the cat's visual cortex. *Journal of Physiology* **195**, 106–54.
2   Coren, S., Ward, L.M. and End, J.T. (1999). *Sensation and Perception*, 5th edn. Harcourt College Publishers, Forth Worth.
3   Treisman, A.M., Cavanagh, P., Fischer, B. and von der Heydt, R. (1990) Form perception and attention: striate cortex and beyond. In: Spillman, L. and Werner, J.S. (eds.) *Visual Perception*. Academic Press, New York.
4   Franks, J. and Brandsford, J. (1971) Abstraction of visual patterns. *Journal of Experimental Psychology* **90**, 65–74.
5   Marr, D. (1982) *Vision*. W.H. Freeman, San Fransisco.

Further reading

Gleitman, H., Fridlund, A.J. and Reisberg, D (1999) *Psychology*, 5th edn. W.W. Norton, New York.
Kanizsa, G. (1976) Subjective contours. *Scientific American* **234**(4), 48–52.

6

Anatomy, Physiology and Pathology of the Skeletal System

Julie Nightingale

Introduction

Successful interpretation of musculo-skeletal plain film images is dependent on an extensive background knowledge of anatomy and physiology, coupled with detailed understanding of the pathophysiology of related injury and disease processes. The first part of this chapter revises and expands upon basic anatomical and physiological concepts related to bones. The reader is referred to supplementary texts where appropriate. Some of the more common bone and joint pathologies are also discussed. The second part covers mechanisms of injury and resulting patterns of trauma seen in both adults and children.

Basic bone anatomy and physiology

The musculo-skeletal system comprises muscle and connective tissues (bone, cartilage, tendons and ligaments). Its primary purpose is locomotion, and it also plays a significant role in protection of vital organs, metabolism of important ions and production of blood cells. The following sections will focus initially on bone tissue from a microscopic and macroscopic perspective. Later bone development, maintenance and homeostasis are also discussed.

Microscopic structure of bone

Bone is a highly vascular connective tissue, its constituent cells being embedded within a three-dimensional **matrix** of collagen and minerals. Bone develops initially from a mesenchyme or cartilage model, whose collagen fibres become permeated with inorganic bone salts, a process

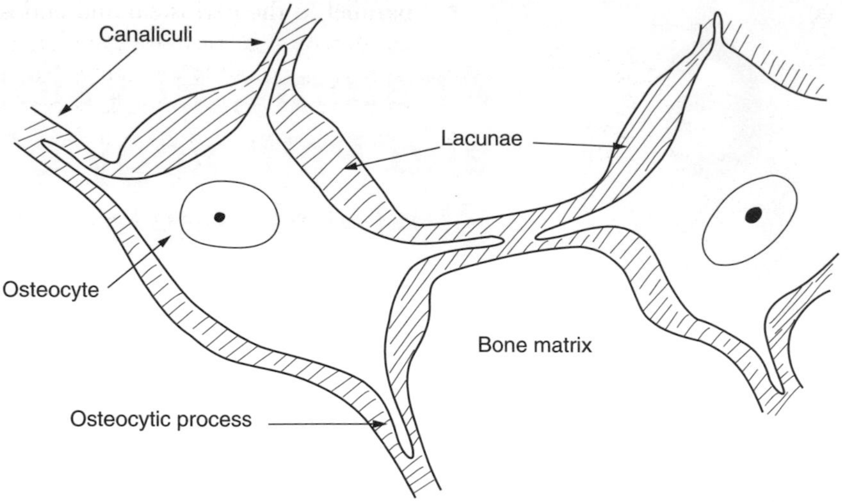

Figure 6.1 Diagram showing the relationship between bone osteocytes.

known as **ossification**. The principal bone salt is hydroxyapatite (primarily calcium and phosphorus), with magnesium, fluoride and citrates also present. These inorganic salts make up approximately 45% of bone tissue mass, with organic tissue such as collagen forming 30%. The remaining 25% is water, mainly found as extracellular fluid within the bone matrix[1]. Hydroxyapatite is highly compression-resistant, whereas the collagen in which it is embedded has high tensile strength. The two combined offer great strength and elasticity (roughly the same principle is used in building work, using a combination of steel and concrete).

Bone cells begin their development as immature stem cells within the bone marrow (**osteoprogenitor cells**), which can metamorphose into active osteoblast or osteoclast cells when required. **Osteoblasts** are collagen-secreting cells, which over time become 'trapped' within their own calcified secretions, forming **osteocytes** (most numerous in young bone tissue). Osteocytes are found within small extracellular fluid-filled spaces called **lacunae**, situated between layers of bone known as **lamellae**. A number of processes extend from the osteocytes into minute channels called **canaliculi**, linking adjacent osteocytes with their vascular network (Figure 6.1). Extracellular fluid is therefore continuous throughout the bone layers, allowing vital nutrients and ions to pass easily to and from the bone cells. **Osteoclasts** are much larger cells than osteoblasts and are less numerous. Their main function is secretion of acidic enzymes (citric and lactic acids and collagenase) to dissolve the bone matrix, so facilitating a balance between bone deposition and removal.

Arrangement of the lamellae

Bone cells and their surrounding matrix are organised within mature layers of tissue called lamellae, situated in the following locations:

Six

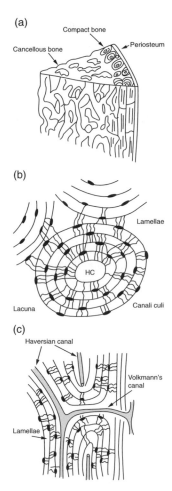

Figure 6.2 Diagram showing the architecture of mature bone. (a) A wedge-shaped cross-section through a long bone. (b) Axial section through compact bone demonstrating layers of concentric bone lamellae (Haversian systems) surrounding a central Haversian canal (HC). (c) Longitudinal section through compact bone, demonstrating linking between Haversian systems via Volkmann's canals.

- parallel to the periosteal and endosteal surfaces of any bone (**circumferential** or **primary** lamellae);
- running in roughly concentric patterns surrounding mature bone vascular channels (**secondary osteons** or **secondary** lamellae);
- lining the crevices between the osteons (**interstitial** lamellae).

The architecture of bone can be seen in Figure 6.2. The secondary osteons are known as **Haversian systems,** and comprise a central canal (carrying blood vessels and nerves) surrounded by between six and fifteen concentric lamellae. Between the lamellae are situated the lacunae, interconnected by a network of canaliculi. The Haversian canals are connected to each other by transverse or obliquely orientated **Volkmann's canals.** Having a mainly longitudinal orientation, Haversian systems give bone high tensile strength that also resists torsional (twisting) and bending forces. The compressive strength of bone is directly related to the amount of transverse fibres, which are most numerous in areas withstanding significant compressive forces (e.g. the ends of weight-bearing long bones). In order to achieve maximum strength and elasticity the lamellae are arranged into very hard, tightly packed tissue called **compact bone,** found on the exterior of all bones. Radiologically compact bone can be seen as a dense, homogeneous radio-opaque tissue forming the external cylinder (**cortex**) of the long bones.

The less well-organised spicules of bone tissue found in the interior surfaces of bone, known as **trabeculae,** often surround a marrow-filled medullary cavity. Superimposed trabeculae create a meshwork of tissue known as **cancellous** or **spongy bone.** It is essentially similar to compact bone, though there is less solid matter and larger bone spaces (i.e. it is more porous). The trabecular pattern is usually aligned along lines of stress within the bone. This fine meshwork pattern can be seen radiographically and is particularly noticeable within the ends of long bones such as the neck of femur.

Table 6.1 summarises the main differences between compact and cancellous bone; however, it is important to note that two other types of

Table 6.1 Comparison of the features of compact and cancellous bone.

	Compact bone	**Cancellous bone**
Alternative names	Lamellar bone Cortical bone	Spongy bone Trabecular bone
Position	External cylinder of long bones (cortex) Thin outer covering of other bones	Interior aspects of small bones Ends (epiphyses) of long bones
Density	Very dense, hard bone	Less dense, porous bone
Structure	Tightly packed, interconnecting Haversian systems (secondary osteons)	Criss-crossed trabeculae with large bone marrow-filled spaces (similar to woven bone)
Properties	Rigidity and strength (resists torsional and bending stresses)	Strength and lightness (resistant to compressive forces)

Six

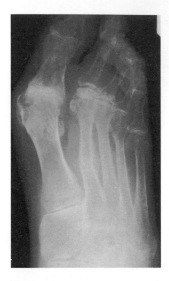

Figure 6.3 Radiograph demonstrating periosteal reaction typical of a stress fracture. The second metatarsal shows the appearance of a raised periosteum on its lateral border, suggesting a metatarsal stress fracture.

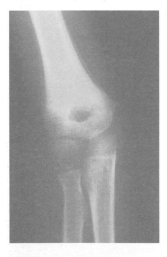

Figure 6.4 Radiograph showing the appearance of a raised periosteum of the paediatric elbow. Paediatric elbow fractures can be subtle, but note the periosteal reaction on both lateral and medial borders of the distal humerus, indicating bleeding from a fracture.

bone tissue may be seen on radiographs. The first is concerned with growth and the healing and repair of fractures, and has a disorganised structure known as **woven bone** or **bone callus**. The second type is known as **osteoid tissue** – this is a non-calcified matrix seen within the immature skeleton prior to ossification, or associated with certain disease processes such as rickets or osteomalacia.

Blood supply and nerves

It is important to appreciate that bone tissue is highly vascular and well innervated. The vascular and nerve supply is intricately connected to the **periosteum**, a thin double membrane surrounding the outer edges of bone. The outer periosteal layer is fibrous and interconnects with tendons and ligaments. The inner layer is elastic and highly vascular, playing a role in nutrition, growth and repair of the underlying bone. The periosteum is thicker and more vascular in immature bones, and gradually thins with age. It cannot be seen radiographically unless there is an underlying pathology (such as a haematoma or infection), which lifts the periosteum away from the cortical bone (Figures 6.3 and 6.4).

There are several discrete points along a bone where the periosteal blood vessels penetrate into the compact bone, the larger nutrient arteries tending to pierce the shaft of long bones obliquely. These entry points may be mistaken for fractures by an untrained observer, but they enter at the same position and always run in the same direction (Figure 6.5). There are numerous smaller vascular foramina within the bone ends (epiphyses) and in small bones.

The bone tissue and cells are supplied via the capillaries of the Haversian canals, with the bone marrow and perichondrium (surrounding the cartilage) also receiving a good supply. However, the blood supply to the articular cartilage within joints, and the epiphyseal cartilage in immature bone, can easily be compromised following trauma. The arteries at either side of a growth plate rarely anastomose, with the **epiphysis** forming a discrete vascular zone in children. In infants and adults the vessels of the diaphysis (shaft) and epiphysis do anastomose, leading to a greater potential for spread of infection or tumour from a long bone through to the joint.

Some bones have a very limited blood supply which can easily be compromised in injury or certain disease processes. In particular the proximal femur and the lunate and scaphoid bone are prone to developing **avascular necrosis** as a sequel to a fracture. Radiographic appearances may show bone sclerosis, cysts and subchondral collapse (Figure 6.6), but may be normal in the early stages. Bone scintigraphy, magnetic resonance imaging or computed tomography are useful in assessing bone necrosis. Large irregular bones such as the innominate bone or scapula receive their superficial supply from the periosteum, but also have nutrient arteries penetrating deep into the cancellous bone. Short bones also receive their supply from the periosteum.

Six

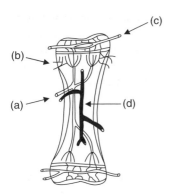

Figure 6.5 The blood supply of a long bone. One or two large diaphyseal nutrient arteries (clear vessels) pierce the shaft obliquely (a), pointing away from the dominant growing end of the bone. Once through the cortex the artery splits into ascending and descending branches. Branching many times, they are joined by metaphyseal (b) and epiphyseal (c) periarticular branches. (Note that in children the growth plate prevents such anastomoses.) Small arterial branches connect with the bone sinusoids which flow into a large central venous sinus (d), or into endosteal canals/Haversian systems. The veins leave the bone alongside the nutrient arteries or pierce the shaft separately.

Nerves are found to be most numerous in the vertebrae, the larger flat bones such as the innominate bone and the skull vault, and in the articular ends of the long bones. The nerves network within the periosteum and then enter into the bone along with the nutrient arteries, the smaller branches travelling alongside the vessels within the Haversian canals.

Classification of bones

There are approximately 206 bones within the adult human skeleton, although the exact number is determined by additional sesamoid bones, vertebrae and ribs in some individuals.

Bones can be classified as long, short, irregular, flat, pneumatic and sesamoid. **Long bones** can be subclassified as **regular** long bones (e.g. the ulna) or **miniature** long bones (e.g. metacarpals and phalanges), although all conform to the same basic pattern. Miniature long bones, however, usually have only one epiphyseal growth plate compared with two in regular bones.

The adult long bone consists of a cylindrical shaft (**diaphysis**) of compact bone (**cortex**) surrounding a medullary cavity filled with yellow bone marrow (Figure 6.7). The cortex thins as it approaches the expanded bone ends (epiphyses), which are filled with cancellous bone and red bone marrow. The articular surfaces of the epiphysis are covered with a layer of radiolucent **hyaline** cartilage. **Periosteum** covers the exterior of the long bones with the exception of the articular surfaces, and **endosteum** (a layer of osteoprogenitor/bone stem cells) lines the internal medullary cavity.

Figure 6.6 Avascular necrosis of both femoral heads. Note the sclerosis of the femoral heads, with a small subchondral fracture and patchy osteolysis in the right hip (b). There is a band-like sclerotic zone in the joint socket, but the cartilage appears intact. Eventually the head may become deformed and flattened.

(a)

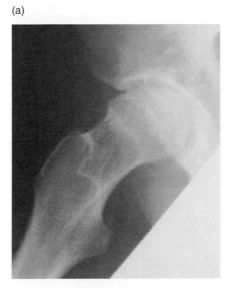

(b)

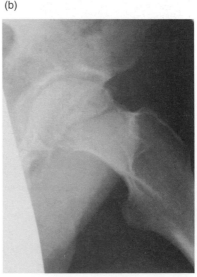

Six

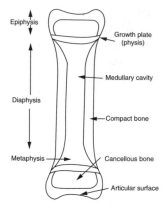

Figure 6.7 The anatomical features of a long bone.

In the young skeleton a zone of growth is evident at the junction of the diaphysis and epiphysis. This epiphyseal **growth plate** or **physis** is also hyaline cartilage and is therefore radiolucent. The actively growing region of the shaft adjacent to the growth plate is termed the **metaphysis**. Following closure of the growth plate, an epiphyseal ridge or line is usually still evident.

Features of bones

Bones vary not only in their primary size and shape but also in their surface features (Table 6.2), which usually develop in post-natal life. The reporting practitioner must be familiar with the gross anatomy of all the individual bones and joints of the skeleton, using standard medical terminology when describing images. Diagrams of individual bones can be found in many texts[2,3].

Development of bone

Ossification begins in early foetal life and is not complete until approximately 25 years of age, when the final growth plates fuse. Ossification

Table 6.2 Features of individual bones.

Feature	Types	Description
Articular surfaces		Parts of the bone forming a joint with neighbouring bone surfaces. These surfaces vary in shape and size dependent upon the range of movement required. Usually smooth and covered with hyaline cartilage
	Facet	Small articular surfaces (e.g. superior articular facets of vertebrae)
	Trochlea	Larger surfaces (pulley-shaped) (e.g. trochlea of distal humerus)
	Condyle	Larger surfaces (knuckle-shaped) (e.g. femoral condyles)
	Head	Expanded proximal ends of long bones (e.g. head of humerus)
Tendon and ligament insertions		Often associated with the articular surfaces, and may be roughened areas, small pits or larger elevations
	Tuberosity, tubercle, trochanter	Large, rough rounded elevations (e.g. greater trochanter of femur)
	Process	Large elevation (e.g. olecranon process of ulna)
	Crest, spine, line	Elongated elevation (e.g. iliac crest)
	Cornu	Curved elevation
	Epicondyles	Small projections adjacent to condyles, primarily for the insertion of ligaments (e.g. distal humerus epicondyles)
Bone depressions and holes	Fossa	Bone depression (e.g. iliac fossa)
	Groove/sulcus	Elongated depression (e.g. bicipital groove)
	Foramen	Small hole in bone (e.g. jugular foramen)
	Canal	Elongated hole or passageway (e.g. auditory canal)
	Aperture	A large hole
	Fissure	Narrow cleft (e.g. superior orbital fissure)
Bone plates	Lamina	A thin plate of bone (e.g. vertebral lamina)

Six

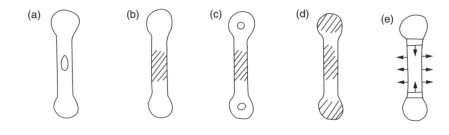

Figure 6.8   The process of endochondral ossification within a long bone begins with a primary ossification centre in the middle of the shaft (a), spreading outwards towards the periphery, where a collar of compact bone begins to form (b). Secondary ossification centres form in the ends of the bones (c), eventually spreading across to form the epiphysis (d). A cartilaginous growth plate remains at the junction of the diaphysis and metaphysis (e). Growth in length continues at the diaphyseal side of the growth plate (metaphysis), while growth in girth is a result of bone being laid down beneath the periosteum.

involves the replacement of a foetal connective tissue template with a mature bone structure. In some cases (notably the skull vault and clavicle) this is a simple process involving the direct replacement of a membrane with bone. This **intramembranous** ossification also occurs within tendons to ossify sesamoid bones. In other bones the process is more complicated, involving a hyaline cartilage template (**endochondral** or **intracartilaginous** ossification) (Figure 6.8).

In both processes the replacement of soft tissue with bone begins within ossification centres which develop within embryonic life, or in foetal life or after birth. Many bones ossify from a single ossification centre (e.g. carpal and tarsal bones, some facial bones) beginning between a timeframe of the eighth week of foetal life until ten years of age. Most bones, however, ossify from several centres. Long bones, for example, have a primary ossification centre within the shaft which develops anywhere between the seventh foetal week and the fifth month of pregnancy, and usually closes around the time of birth. The ends of the long bones (epiphyses) are still cartilaginous at birth, but begin to develop secondary ossification centres from birth to the late teens. Larger epiphyses tend to ossify first. Between the primary and secondary ossification centres a cartilaginous growth plate persists, eventually fusing to create epiphyseal lines seen on the surface of mature bone. Interpretation of paediatric radiographic images can be problematic when faced with several ossification centres at different stages of development (Figure 6.9). Knowledge of the timing of ossification and fusion of the growth plates within different bones will assist in the interpretation. Some texts offer standard tables and images of skeletal maturity[4,5] but it is important to recognise that the data are usually based upon research on well-nourished white children. Some subtle differences between races do exist, and ossification tends to occur earlier in females than in males due to the actions of oestrogens at puberty. Mnemonics have been developed to assist in learning the order of ossification in different bony sites (see CRITOL in Chapter 7, pp. 145–7).

A number of generalised disorders of skeletal ossification and development (bone dysplasias) are seen in clinical practice, and they may be congenital/hereditary or acquired (in the case of deficiencies). These dysplasias typically have characteristic image appearances and may be classified as affecting predominantly the epiphysis, the metaphysis or the

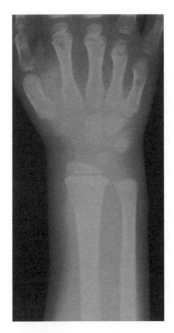

Figure 6.9   An incomplete fracture of the distal radius. Note that seven of the carpal bones are in different stages of ossification.

Six

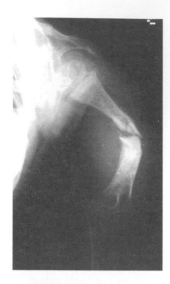

Figure 6.10 Osteogenesis imperfecta (congenital). Widespread osteoporosis, with bowing of the long bones and widened metaphyses. This brittle bone condition has led to a pathological fracture of the humerus. Numerous other fractures were noted post-partum.

spine. Examples include syndromes leading to dwarfism (e.g. achondroplasia and the mucopolysaccharidoses), and those that are characterised by abnormalities of bone density (e.g. osteopoikilosis and osteopetrosis). Some dysplasias have a particularly poor prognosis, including congenital osteogenesis imperfecta (Figure 6.10). This condition is characterised by a defect in collagen synthesis which inhibits bone production. Bones are osteoporotic and fragile, and in some types of this disease neonates acquire multiple fractures *in utero* and post-partum.

Endochondral growth

The actively growing region of a long bone is the metaphysis, which is responsible for the increase in length of a bone (the increase in girth of a bone is largely attributed to the laying down of new bone beneath the periosteum). Most long bones have growth plates at either end of the diaphysis, and microscopically they show highly organised layers of **chondrocytes** (cartilaginous cells). The chondrocytes undergo changes as they traverse the layers, with cells closest to the diaphysis being older and undergoing rapid growth. The different layers are explained in the flow chart in Figure 6.11 and accompanying diagram (Figure 6.12).

Fractures traversing the immature growth plate will attain greater significance if they interfere with the proliferating zone, as they are likely to result in growth arrest. This may not be particularly significant for a metacarpal growth plate injury, but may have enormous consequences for growth arrest within a lower limb bone.

Remodelling

The original connective tissue template is only a rough approximation of the final bony form, and requires regular readjustment (remodelling) to adapt to stresses such as weight bearing. Bone remodelling continues throughout life, and requires a constant shift between bone reabsorption (breakdown) and deposition by the osteocytes. This process is most evident when activity levels change dramatically, but even with normal activity levels remodelling is necessary. This is because **microfractures** occur within the trabeculae as a normal side-effect of general wear and tear, and worn-out osteocytes also need replacing. Remodelling is perhaps most notable during fracture healing and repair.

Bone maintenance and homeostasis

Bone maintenance is dependent upon the correct intake and metabolism of calcium, phosphorus and certain vitamins, and is under the influence

Six

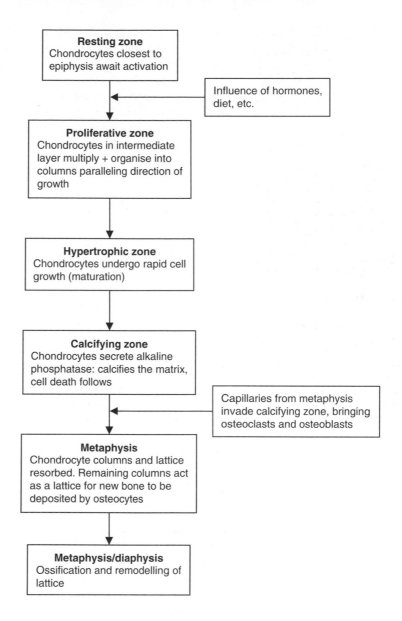

Figure 6.11 Flow chart demonstrating the function of chondrocytes across the growth plate.

of a range of hormones. Bone plays an essential part in the homeostasis of blood and tissue **calcium levels** (Figure 6.13). In the presence of **parathormone** (parathyroid hormone or PTH), approximately 1% of bone calcium is available to be quickly released from bone tissue into the bloodstream[6].

Low levels of circulating calcium cause an elevation of PTH, which in turn indirectly increases osteoclastic function. Osteoclasts secrete acidic enzymes (citric and lactic acid and collagenase) to 'dissolve' bone and release calcium from the hydroxyapatite crystals. At the same time PTH

Six

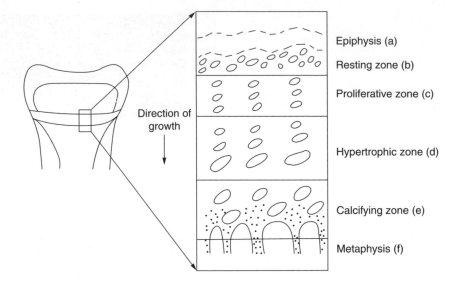

Figure 6.12 The functional zones of the growth plate. A cross-section through the growth plate has been magnified to demonstrate the zones of resting chondrocytes (b), chondrocyte mitosis (c), growth (d), calcification (e) and eventual lysis, ossification and remodelling (f).

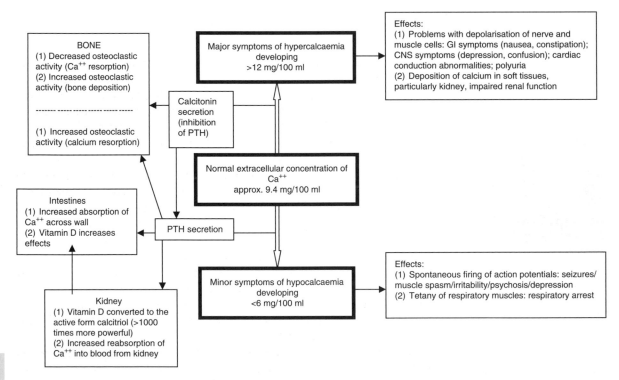

Figure 6.13 The role of bone in the homeostasis of blood calcium levels. PTH, parathyroid hormone; GI, gastrointestinal; CNS, central nervous system.

Six

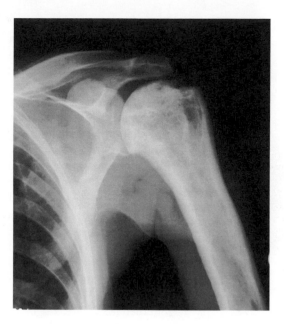

Figure 6.14 Paget's disease of the proximal humerus. Abnormal remodelling of bone (with simultaneous osteoblastic and osteoclastic activity) has led to bone sclerosis and thickening, with an osteolytic focus within the greater tuberosity.

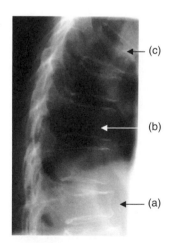

Figure 6.15 Osteoporotic changes in the thoracolumbar spine. Note the anterior wedging (a), the loss of density coupled with thinning and accentuation of the cortices (b), and the possible compression fracture (c).

also causes the renal tubules to reabsorb more calcium, and the bowel wall to increase the absorption of calcium into the bloodstream. All of these factors work together to raise the circulating calcium levels. Abnormal long-term influence of PTH causes an excess of osteoclastic activity, releasing too much calcium into the bloodstream. This results in overactivity of both osteoclasts and osteoblasts, leading to widespread **bone erosions** and **osteitis fibrosa**.

When calcium levels become high, **calcitonin** is secreted from the thyroid gland. This hormone suppresses the level of activity of the osteoclasts, thus reducing the available calcium. Although calcitonin opposes PTH, the overall effects are not as important. However, because calcitonin suppresses osteoclastic activity, it may be used as a therapeutic agent to counter bone loss in both Paget's disease (Figure 6.14) and osteoporosis (Figure 6.15). Osteoporosis is characterised by a generalised loss of bone mineral, causing an increased fragility of bone. The aetiology of osteoporosis is complex, but it may be influenced by a dietary deficiency of calcium or of **vitamin D** (cholecalciferol), which will also affect circulating calcium levels.

Vitamin D (more a hormone than a vitamin) is found in certain foods and is also produced as a skin response to the ultraviolet rays in sunlight, but its effects are minimal until it is converted into its activated form calcitriol by the renal tubules. At normal levels its actions increase the intestinal absorption of calcium and promote bone deposition. At higher levels (with PTH) it promotes bone reabsorption. In some ethnic groups vitamin D deficiency has been a problem, but in an effort to improve child health it is now added to certain food products such as

Six

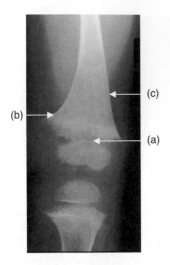

(c)

(b)

(a)

Figure 6.16 Rickets. Predominant features include a widened lucent calcifying zone of the growth plates (containing unmineralised osteoid tissue) (a); widened, irregular, cupped metaphyses (b); bowing of the femur caused by weight bearing (c).

flour. A prolonged deficiency of vitamin D in children will result in a major disturbance of growth cartilage and ossification, causing the characteristic osteopenia and 'bowing' deformities of the extremities seen in **rickets** (Figure 6.16). In adults a prolonged deficiency will result in **osteomalacia**, a condition characterised by poorly mineralised osteoid tissue. This condition is occasionally seen following multiple pregnancies or malnutrition. Calcitriol may be administered therapeutically to counteract calcium imbalances associated with hypothyroidism or chronic renal failure.

Other vitamins are also important in normal growth and maintenance of the skeletal system. **Vitamin C** (ascorbic acid) promotes the normal development of growth cartilages and the metaphyses and, although rare, a deficiency can lead to poor bone and connective tissue growth, weakness and fractures (the disease must be longstanding for radiographic signs to develop). The condition is known as **scurvy**, mainly affecting infants who have been fed on boiled or pasteurised milk (boiling destroys vitamin C). An excess of **vitamin A** in infants will also result in thin growth plates, premature maturation of the skeleton, and bulging of the fontanelles, whereas a deficiency will lead to growth retardation, particularly of the skull base. (This can lead to narrow skull foramina, with resultant compression of nerves and vessels.)

Growth and development are also influenced by the following hormones.

- **Thyroxine** from the thyroid gland influences the rate of body metabolism. It is responsible for effective remodelling and the mature shape of bones.
- Hormones secreted from the ovaries, testes and adrenal glands influence the rate of growth and the state of maturity. **Oestrogen** is particularly influential – in excess it leads to an increased bone growth, such as the growth spurts at puberty. When deficient (particularly in relation to the onset of the menopause) osteoporosis will occur, resulting in a reduction in the overall quantity of bone tissue. This is because oestrogen prevents the differentiation of monocytes into osteoclasts, therefore a deficiency leads to an increase in osteoclasts, with resultant net bone loss.
- **Human growth hormone** (**HGh**) from the anterior lobe of the pituitary gland controls normal growth and the cessation of growth (i.e. the closure of the growth plates). An excess of HGh will lead to **gigantism** in children and **acromegaly** in adults. Acromegaly is often associated with pituitary adenomas leading to an overproduction of HGh after the growth plates of the long bones have fused. This leads to some bones increasing in width, particularly noticeable being the enlarging hands, feet and mandible. A deficiency of HGh may lead to **pituitary dwarfism** or short-statured children. Short stature (approximately 1 in 5000) may also be a result of genetic influences, and it is sometimes treated with additional HGh.

Six

Bone pathology

When assessing trauma radiographs, the reporting practitioner should be aware of a range of bone pathologies that could be either incidental (but nonetheless important) findings, or implicated in the mechanism of injury (pathological fracture). As outlined above, problems with bone metabolism will usually result in a net loss of bone (**osteopenia**), although occasionally irregular or excessive bone deposition can occur (**hyperostosis**). A full discussion of pathological conditions affecting bone is beyond the scope of this book, but a brief outline of the more commonly encountered metabolic and endocrine disorders is given in Table 6.3.

Whereas the metabolic disorders are often generalised, bone tumours are usually localised (with the exception of multiple myeloma and metastases). Once a lesion has been recognised, the practitioner will usually be able to arrive at a diagnosis based on the plain film findings, many of which are pathognomic for particular lesions. If a diagnosis cannot be made with certainty, then the practitioner must place the lesion in one of the following categories outlined by Manaster[7].

- A benign lesion which is best ignored (e.g. fibrous cortical defect).
- A lesion which is most probably benign, but should be followed up by interval radiographs to confirm the diagnosis (e.g. non-ossifying fibroma).
- A benign symptomatic lesion which requires surgery (e.g. osteoid osteoma).
- A lesion requiring follow-up studies to determine benign or malignant status (e.g. chondroma).
- A malignant lesion requiring further imaging and/or biopsy (e.g. Ewing's tumour, Figure 6.17).

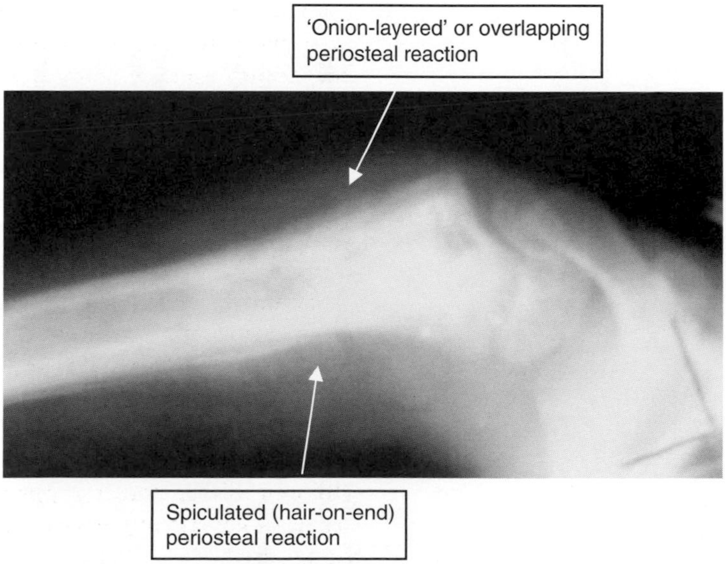

'Onion-layered' or overlapping periosteal reaction

Spiculated (hair-on-end) periosteal reaction

Figure 6.17 Ewing's sarcoma in the proximal humerus of a young child. Note the characteristic 'onion skin' and spiculated periosteal reaction, and occluded medullary cavity.

Six

Six

Table 6.3 Features of selected bone pathologies resulting from metabolic, hormonal and dietary disturbances.

Pathology	Region	Radiographic appearance	Notes
Osteoporosis	Vertebrae and distal forearm (type 1) Hips, proximal humerus, pelvis (type 2)	Uniform decrease in bone density (osteopenia) with accentuation of primary trabeculae (especially femoral neck) and thinning bone cortex The bone is normal histologically Insufficiency fractures of spine and hip Wedge-shaped vertebral deformities (dorsal spine) Colles # of distal radius	Type 1: post-menopausal women >50 years Type 2: Both sexes over 75 years Other causes include: endocrine (hyperparathyroidism, Cushing's disease, hyperthyroidism, pregnancy), medications (corticosteroids), malnutrition (scurvy, calcium deficiency), oophorectomy Radiographic changes seen after 30–50% bone mass is lost. Calculation of bone mineral density essential for accurate assessment (e.g. dual energy X-ray absorptiometry)
Regional osteoporosis	Any region, particularly extremities and hip	Diffuse, patchy osteopenia, restricted to a particular region	Usually caused by immobilisation (disuse osteoporosis) Transient regional osteoporosis (e.g. hip)
Hyperparathyroidism	Resorption of mainly cortical bone from multiple areas: phalangeal tufts pelvic SI joints and pubic symphysis knee and spine epiphyses occasionally tiny osteopenic lesions in skull (PA hand most effective for serial follow-up)	Bone resorption underlying periosteum, cartilage, endosteal, etc. Crystal deposits (e.g. urates) Regional osteosclerosis (e.g. vertebral bodies) Multiple or solitary Brown's tumours (osteoclastoma) Soft tissue calcification	Variable clinical findings as many organs may be involved (e.g. liver, kidney, parathyroids). Three main types: primary: Parathyroid overgrowth or adenomas (87%), leading to elevated PTH levels (often asymptomatic) secondary: Chronic hypocalcaemia caused by malabsorption syndromes or renal failure leading to excessive PTH levels tertiary: Follows longstanding secondary hyperparathyroidism, where parathyroids begin to oversecrete leading to hypercalcaemia
Osteomalacia	Widespread involvement	Decreased density (osteopenia) and accentuation and widening of trabeculae Thickening of long bones Bilateral transverse insufficiency fractures and Looser's zones (radiolucent bands of poorly healing fractures)	Mature bone osteoid is poorly mineralised, caused by: vitamin D deficiency: inadequate exposure to UV light, malabsorption syndromes, inadequate intake, abnormal metabolism. liver/kidney disease (reduces effectiveness of vitamin D) some drugs, e.g. anticonvulsants (affect PTH secretion)
Rickets	Appendicular skeleton, particularly proximal	Generalised growth retardation and small stature	An abnormality of mineralisation of the growth plate, with similar causes to

Condition	Distribution	Radiographic features	Comments
	humerus, distal radius, and around knees. Metaphyseal involvement	Osteopenia, particularly in the calcifying zone of the metaphyses. Bowing deformity of long bones, scoliosis and vertebral body deformity. Widening and irregularities of the growth plates, with 'cupping' of the metaphysis	osteomalacia. Infants can present with tetany or convulsions, skull deformities and thickening of joints
Renal osteodystrophy	Generalised	Range of appearances, including prominent osteosclerosis, and signs of osteomalacia/rickets and secondary hyperparathyroidism	Most have known chronic renal insufficiency, resulting in interference with calcium metabolism and vitamin D activation
Hypoparathyroidism	Generalised or localised (spine and hands)	Osteosclerosis. Soft tissue calcification, particularly subcutaneous and basal ganglia. Hypoplastic dentition. Some types show osteoporosis, and increased density in metaphyses and vertebral endplates	Deficiency of PTH production, usually following surgical resection of parathyroids. Patient may have neuromuscular disorders caused by hypocalcaemia
Scurvy	Sites of rapid growth, including ends of long bones (especially knee), and costochondral junction	Radiographic signs seen only in longstanding disease states: subperiosteal haemorrhage and periostitis; transverse radio-opaque zone of proliferation; transverse radiolucent line in metaphysis; widespread epiphyseal osteoporosis	Rare vitamin C deficiency causing abnormal collagen formation, seen in: infants over 6 months fed boiled or pasteurised milk, which destroys vitamin C (infantile scurvy); elderly patients who are malnourished
Hypothyroidism	Generalised	Osteopenia. Delayed skeletal development, including epiphyseal deformity. Slipped femoral epiphyses. Erosive arthritis. Calcifications and crystal deposition. Widened disc spaces (spine)	The thyroid secretes hormones which control basal metabolic rate, controlling cardiac and neurological function. Deficient secretion is caused by thyroid failure or pituitary/hypothalamic disease. Dry skin and hair, lethargy, oedema, cold intolerance, weight gain, paraesthesia
Hyperthyroidism	Generalised	Osteopathy. Osteoporosis. Accelerated skeletal maturity	Thyrotoxicosis from overproduction of thyroid hormone, caused by Graves' disease or thyroid adenomas. Nervousness, palpitations and tachycardia, fatigue, dyspnoea, goitre, frequency of bowel movements, eye problems, etc.

Six

Table 6.3 *Continued*

Pathology	Region	Radiographic appearance	Notes
Paget's disease	Generalised, but skull, pelvis and vertebral bodies most common May affect limbs	Affected bones are thickened and bent (particularly lower limbs), plus spine kyphosis Trabeculae are coarse and sparse, giving a honeycomb appearance Density may be increased or decreased Pathological fractures common	Unknown cause, but possibly a viral connection. Common in the over-50s in Britain, Australia and Germany Alternating bone formation and resorption, causing irregular thickening (and weakening) of the cortices and trabeculae Where bone resorption predominates, bones are easily bowed. Where formation predominates, bones become very brittle and easily fractured
Acromegaly (hyperpituitarism)	Skull, mandible and soft tissue changes	Enlargement of mandible, phalanges, sella turcica, joints and disc spaces Thickening of long bones and skull, with early degenerative disease (e.g. osteophytes) Enlargement of vertebral bodies with ossification of anterior discs	Hypersecretion of growth hormone after closure of the growth plates, caused by anterior pituitary adenomas Selective enlargement of skeleton and soft tissues (e.g. tongue, palms and soles), menstrual problems, headaches, increased metabolic rate, weight gain, arthropathies
Gigantism (hyperpituitarism)	Generalised, with entire skeleton affected proportionally	Symmetrical overgrowth of all skeletal and soft tissues	As above, except the hypersecretion occurs in children, prior to closure of growth plates
Short stature (hypopituitarism)	Generalised and proportional slow growth, or complex growth pattern (Frohlich's)	Reduced growth of all tissues in children: epiphyses unfused epiphyseal slipping at knee and hip	Caused by hyposecretion of growth hormone: proportionate dwarfism, due to growth retardation delayed skeletal maturation, coupled with hypogonadism and obesity (Frohlich's syndrome)
Calcium pyrophosphate dihydrate (CPPD) disease	Intra-articular crystal deposition: knee, wrist, metacarpophalangeal joints	Often chondrocalcinosis (cartilage calcification, especially knee menisci/cartilage) Soft tissue swelling Subchondral cysts and sclerosis	Relatively common disorder of middle age/elderly May be associated with other disorders such as gout or hypoparathyroidism

Other conditions:
Fluorosis
Hypervitaminosis A
Hypervitaminosis D

SI, sacroiliac; PA, postero-anterior; PTH, parathyroid hormone.

Six

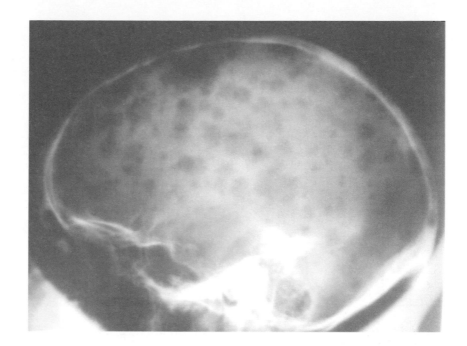

Figure 6.18 Bone metastases from a breast cancer primary: multiple lytic lesions representing a 'moth-eaten' pattern. The lesions have a poorly defined zone of transition, no sclerotic margin and no periosteal reaction. However some metastases may be sclerotic, particularly from a prostate primary.

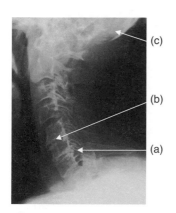

(c)

(b)

(a)

Figure 6.19 Degenerative changes in the cervical spine, including the presence of osteophytes (a) and joint space narrowing (b). However note also the more sinister pathology – there is cortical destruction of the occiput, which is a metastasis (c).

Bone metastases (Figures 6.18 and 6.19) are more common than primary tumours of bone (Figures 6.20 and 6.21). Table 6.4 outlines the features of the more commonly encountered bone tumours.

Inflammatory conditions of the skeletal system are, like tumours, generally localised to a particular bone or joint, and may be acute, subacute or chronic (Table 6.5). Osteomyelitis occurs when pathogens (usually blood-borne bacteria such as *Staphylococcus aureus*) infiltrate the bone marrow and damage local tissue, spreading quickly to the bone tissue. Osteomyelitis may produce characteristic radiographic patterns, including elevation of the periosteum caused by a build-up of blood and oedema fluid (particularly in children), and the presence of sequestra (dead bone tissue) (Figures 6.22 and 6.23). The condition can appear very aggressive, simulating malignant tumour.

Osteomyelitis may be in an epiphyseal location in infants, but is usually metaphyseal in children (as the lack of anastomosing blood vessels helps prevent the spread of infection across the growth plate). In adults a diaphyseal lesion can easily spread to involve the joint cavity, resulting in a septic arthritis (Figure 6.24).

Six

Table 6.4   Key features of bone tumours.

Type	Region	Features	Radiographic appearance
Simple bone cyst (benign, not really a tumour)	Usually proximal femur, tibia or humerus	Usually children up to 15 years Disappear spontaneously Pathological fractures common	Translucent region in metaphysis or diaphysis Expanded bone with thin cortex Similar to a fibrous cortical defect (filled with fibrous tissue rather than fluid)
Aneurysmal bone cyst (benign vascular lesion)	Metaphyses of long bones, spine, pelvis	Expansile, highly vascular lesion Blood-filled cavities May be associated with other lesions (e.g. giant cell tumour), or follow trauma Age 10–30 years	Large, expansile, lytic metaphyseal lesion Often excentric position Often rapid growth and involvement of soft tissue, mimics malignancy
Osteoid osteoma (benign bone tumour)	Usually femur or tibia (cortex), or posterior elements of spinal column	Small, round or oval tumour (nidus) <2 cm wide Contains osteoid (new bone) surrounded by dense bone <30 years	Small central lucent area (nidus) surrounded by dense sclerosis Appearances similar to Brodie's abscess
Multiple myeloma (malignant marrow tumour)	Found in areas of red marrow: axial skeleton, proximal humerus/hip	Most common bone neoplasm Usually multiple lesions, but may present as a large single lesion (plasmocytoma) Age 45–65 years Proliferation of plasma cells in bone marrow which spreads to cortex	Multiple 'punched-out' lucent lesions in more than one bone May be generalised osteoporosis with compression fractures
Osteosarcoma (malignant bone tumour)	Metaphyses of long bones, esp. humerus, distal femur and proximal tibia	Males (2:1), commonly 10–20 years Most common malignant bone tumour Fibrous dysplasia/Paget's disease or post-irradiation may be precursors in older people (over 50) Pain and swelling, usually acute and aggressive course Spreads readily to the lungs Resistant to chemotherapy, therefore generally poor prognosis	Destructive lesion with a 'moth-eaten' appearance Spiculated periosteal reaction: streaks of soft tissue calcification known as the 'sunburst' appearance Soft tissue mass, and early myositis ossificans Periosteal new bone at the margins of the mass
Chondrosarcoma (malignant cartilage tumour)	Flat bones, esp. pelvis and scapula	40–60 years 25% of sarcomas: malignant tumour of cartilage Pain and swelling, indolent (slow) growth Poor response to chemotherapy Tumours large on presentation	Destructive medullary lobular lesions with mottled, punctate or annular calcification Difficult to distinguish from benign cartilage lesions (e.g. chondroma) May begin as an exostosis, and is surrounded by flecks of calcification

Six

Tumour	Location	Features	Radiological appearance
Ewing's sarcoma (malignant marrow tumour)	Diaphyses of long bones Flat bones	10–20 years Neuroectodermal tumour (embryological origin) Widespread metastases in lungs, other bones and bone marrow Good response to chemotherapy	Soft tissue mass/bone destruction with overlapping periosteal reaction (onion-skin appearance) (see Figure 6.17 p. 75)
Chondroma/enchondroma (benign cartilage tumour)	Long bones and miniature long bones of foot and hand	May be single or multiple Must be differentiated from a simple bone cyst or chondrosarcoma Age 30–40 years	Well-defined lucent area in medullary cavity, with cortical thinning/expansion May be flecks of calcification
Osteochondroma/exostosis (benign cartilage tumour)	Metaphysis of long bones	Most common primary tumour Adolescents, tumour usually stops growing when growth plate fuses Cartilaginous overgrowth of growth plate which later ossifies May be single or multiple	Mushroom-shaped or conical outgrowths extending from the metaphysis May be multiple (hereditary)
Metastatic bone tumours (Figure 6.18, p. 79)	Axial skeleton, femur and proximal humerus (80%)	Much more common than primary bone tumours, occur in over 25% of extraskeletal malignancy Spread from prostate and breast, but also from gastro-intestinal tract, kidney and lungs 50–70 years approx.	Destructive lytic lesions (moth-eaten bone) In prostate metastases the deposits may be sclerotic Generalised osteoporosis (see Figure 6.15 p. 73)
Giant cell tumour or osteoclastoma (benign or malignant tumour—uncertain origin)	Epiphyseal cancellous bone, particularly around knee or wrist	May be benign, locally invasive or malignant Occurs in mature bone after growth plates have fused, usually 20–40 years Large tumours abutting joint margins Contains multinucleated giant cells	Asymmetrically placed lucent area in the epiphysis Cortex thins and may break (see Figure 6.21 p. 83)
Non-ossifying fibroma (NOF)/Benign fibrous cortical defect (BFCD) (benign fibrous lesions)	Long bones of lower limb, ulna	5–20 years Cortically based lesion of the metaphysis Probably not neoplasms, but begin as a growth plate defect Asymptomatic lesions, which probably heal spontaneously	Oval lesion situated in cortex of metaphysis <2cm (BFCD) or >2cm (NOF) Lytic lesion with sclerotic border

Six

Table 6.5 Key features of bone and joint infections.

Type	Organism and route of spread	Features	Radiographic appearance
Septic (pyogenic/infectious) arthritis	75% Gram + cocci, e.g. *Staphylococcus aureus*, streptococcus Haematogenic seeding (blood), direct (wounds, arthroscopy and per-operative)	Common in intravenous drug abusers, joint surgery, the immunocompromised (often opportunistic infections), infancy Often large joints, esp. hip and knee, exhibit swelling, pain, heat	Adult: rapid effusion and joint space narrowing, osteoporosis around the joint, destruction of subchondral bone with erosions. Sclerotic reaction and later ankylosis Child: swelling, subluxation or dislocation of ossification centre, metaphyseal osteomyelitis, joint space narrowing X-rays may be normal for up to three weeks
Acute osteomyelitis	*S. aureus* most common, but also streptococcus (young children) *Pseudomonas*, *Brucella*, *Escherichia coli*, etc. Haematogenic spread, or direct from adjacent tissue or a wound	Usually children, but common in diabetics, IV drug abusers and immunocompromised Usually metaphyses of long bones and spine, epiphyses in infants. Spine and small bones in adults Pain in limb for up to 3 months with no fever, or acute onset in children (fever, lethargy, heat)	Plain radiographic appearances are not visible for at least 10 days. Radionuclide imaging studies may be positive within two days Blurring of soft tissue fat planes, followed by poorly differentiated bone cortical destruction and periosteal reaction Sequestra (necrotic bone islands) may develop Slipped epiphyses and growth deformity may result in infants
Chronic osteomyelitis	As above. Some organisms more resistant to antibiotic therapy (e.g. *Pseudomonas*, *Enterobacter*)	With prompt treatment, <5% should go on to develop the chronic form May require drainage and surgical debridement, long-term antibiotics and bone grafts	Osteosclerosis and cortical thickening Periosteal thickening and excess bone deposition Ill-defined lytic lesions and sequestra (separated pieces/islands of bone)
Brodie's abscess	Staphylococcal organisms Subacute osteomyelitis	Subacute osteomyelitis Usually children Usually distal tibial metaphysis	Circular, well-circumscribed lytic lesion with a sclerotic margin (similar to osteoid osteoma) Metaphyseal region Channel may communicate with the growth plate

(a) (b)

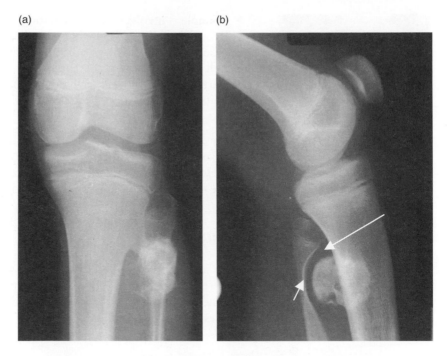

Figure 6.20 Osteochondroma of the tibial metaphysis. The cauliflower-shaped cartilaginous tumour extends from a small stalk. Note that the fibula has deviated (arrows) but has not been infiltrated by the lesion, indicating a slow-growing, benign course.

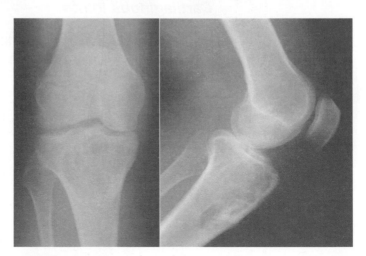

Figure 6.21 Giant cell tumour of the proximal tibia extending to the articular surfaces of the epiphysis, seen on antero-posterior (AP) and lateral aspects. In children the lesion is metaphyseal, as the growth plate hinders progression into the epiphysis.

Anatomy and classification of joints

A joint or **articulation** is formed at the junction of two or more adjacent bones. The anatomy of different joints varies considerably, influencing both the range of motion and joint stability. Knowledge of the specific anatomy of individual joints (including the associated ligaments, tendons, bursae and muscles) is essential for an informed interpretation of trauma radiographs. On the basis of complexity joints may be termed as follows.

Six

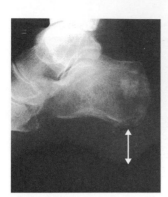

Figure 6.22 Acute osteomalacia of the calcaneum. Note the patchy osteosclerosis and the extensive soft tissue swelling in the heel pad (arrow).

- **Simple** – involves two articulating surfaces, where one is usually concave and one is convex (e.g. the interphalangeal joints).
- **Compound** – involves more than two articular surfaces (e.g. the elbow joint, where the capitulum and trochlea of the humerus articulate with the radius and ulna).
- **Complex** – involves articular discs or menisci (e.g. the wrist or knee joint).

Joints were formerly classified according to the degree of motion permitted, and included non-movable, slightly movable and freely movable joints. However, this has now been replaced by a classification based on the type of connective tissue associated with the joint.

Fibrous joints

Fibrous joints are connected by fibrous tissue. They have no joint cavity and therefore are immovable. Examples include the **sutures** of the skull vault, the joints between the radius and ulna, and tibia and fibula (**syndesmoses**), and the **gomphoses** (tooth peg sockets).

Cartilaginous joints

Cartilaginous joints permit a small degree of movement and include joints united by hyaline cartilage (**synchondroses**) such as the costal car-

Figure 6.23 A purulent osteomyelitis in the tibia of a child. The majority of the diaphysis is involved, but the epiphyses are spared. The chequered appearance results from inflammatory osteolysis and reactive bone sclerosis. There is extensive periosteal reaction and calcification. A large osteomyelitic focus appears to house a sequestrum (arrow).

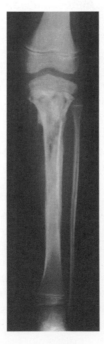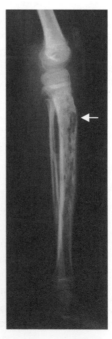

Six

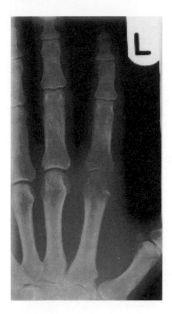

Figure 6.24 Septic arthritis in the second metacarpophalangeal joint. Note the periarticular osteoporosis (caused by an increased blood supply), the decreased joint space (caused by cartilage destruction), and early signs of bone destruction around the joint space.

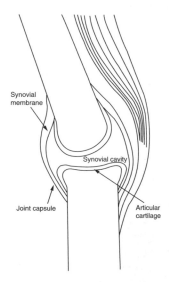

Figure 6.25 Longitudinal section of a typical synovial joint.

tilages of the ribs and sternum, and the 'temporary' epiphyseal growth plates. Cartilaginous joints also include those united by fibrocartilage (called **symphyses**) such as the pelvic symphysis pubis. This joint normally permits very limited movement, though during pregnancy the circulating hormones allow the cartilage to soften and the joint to stretch, allowing a wider pelvic canal for parturition. (It is interesting to note that the same maternal hormones can also cause softening and stretching of some of the foetal joints, especially the hip.) The intervertebral joints of the spine are also symphyses, allowing very limited movement between opposing vertebrae – although the combined effect of all of these joints results in a mobile vertebral column.

Synovial joints

Synovial joints contain synovial fluid and allow a wide range of movement. Such joints are more complex than fibrous and cartilaginous joints, but they all have a basic structure as shown in Figure 6.25. The articulating surfaces of the bone are covered by a thin layer of **articular hyaline cartilage** (between 1 mm and 5 mm thick), creating a smooth surface and moulding the joint. Young cartilage is shiny and bluish-white in colour, but it thins and yellows with age. The cartilage is effectively similar to a sponge, being able to soak up joint fluid when at rest, which then seeps out when the cartilage is compressed during use. Some joints also have additional **articular discs**, helping to deepen the joint cavity and provide additional support.

The joint cavity is enclosed in a **joint capsule**, which helps to bind the bones together. The capsule has an outer layer of fibrous tissue continuous with the periosteum of the bones and in places this can thicken to form **ligaments**. The inner layer of the capsule is a **synovial membrane**, which lines the joint throughout except the articular cartilage. This membrane produces **synovial fluid**, a mixture of proteins, polysaccharides, fat and cells, essentially similar to blood serum. The main polysaccharide is hyaluronic acid, contributing a 'slippery' consistency to the fluid, which lubricates the joint surfaces.

Some synovial joints are more complex, and the synovial membrane may extend for some distance away from the joint, creating a sack-like **bursa**. Bursae are usually found in areas of compression where adjacent structures would otherwise create friction, such as between tendons and bone.

Nerves and blood vessels do not enter the joint cavity but are associated with the fibrous capsule and to a lesser extent the synovial membrane. The articular cartilage obtains nourishment from the underlying cancellous bone, the synovial fluid, and from a network of small vessels at the margins of the cartilage.

There are a number of different types of synovial joint as seen in Table 6.6, those with a high degree of mobility such as the ball and socket joint usually having lower stability (and therefore are more prone to disloca-

Six

Table 6.6   Features of synovial joints.

Type of joint	Anatomical description	Movement(s) permitted	Examples
Hinge	Closely moulded surfaces (similar to the hinge of a door). Sides of joints are strengthened by very strong ligaments	Forwards and backwards swing (uni-axial/planar movement) with a small degree of rotation	Elbow (humero-ulnar joint) Interphalangeal joints
Plane	Flat articular surfaces, with a slight curvature	Sliding of one bone on another	Intermetatarsal joints Some intercarpal joints
Condylar	Surfaces formed by two distinct convex condyles which articulate with two concave surfaces. The two surfaces can be in separate joint cavities (as in the temporomandibular joints)	Uni-axial, but a limited amount of rotation in a second plane	Knee joint Temporomandibular joints
Pivot	Central bony pivot surrounded by a ring of bone and ligaments	Uni-planar with rotation around a stationary central pivot (radial head within the radial notch of humerus) Ring may rotate around a stationary pivot (arch of C1 around a stationary odontoid peg (dens) of C2)	Atlanto-axial joint (C1/C2) Radial head/humeral joint
Ellipsoid	A convex oval surface articulates with a concave elliptical surface	Bi-planar (movement at right angles to each other)	Radiocarpal joint Metacarpophalangeal joints
Ball and socket	A spherical or egg-shaped head articulates with a cup-like concavity	Multi-planar, with movement in all three planes	Shoulder (glenohumeral) joint Hip joint
Saddle joint	Opposing surfaces are concavoconvex. Convexity of larger surface opposed with concavity of the smaller	Bi-planar movements at right angles often with associated small degrees of rotation of the bones	First carpometacarpal joint (thumb) Ankle joint Calcaneocuboid joint

tion and subluxation). In order to increase stability a number of anatomical adaptations are found in some joints, including the muscles of the rotator cuff mechanism in the glenohumeral (shoulder) joint, the fibrocartilaginous labra in the hip and shoulder, and the extremely strong capsule and extra-articular ligaments in the hip. The knee, a modified hinge joint, is strengthened and stabilised by adaptations including the semicircular menisci that deepen the joint surface, and the two intra-articular cruciate ligaments which prevent hyperextension and posterior displacement of the tibia. The knee joint is further strengthened by extra-articular ligaments and the tendons of the thigh muscles.

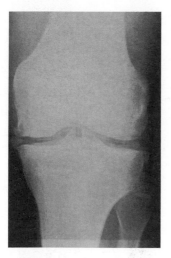

Figure 6.26
Chondrocalcinosis, caused by CPPD disease. Inorganic crystals are laid down in the menisci and articular cartilage, resulting in their calcification.

Joint disease

A number of conditions affecting joints can be an incidental finding on trauma radiographs, with productive disorders such as osteoarthritis at one end of the spectrum and erosive disorders such as rheumatoid arthritis at the other end. Many other joint disorders such as the crystal deposition syndromes, which include gout and calcium pyrophosphate dihydrate crystal deposition (CPPD disease) (Figure 6.26), lie somewhere in the middle of the spectrum. The most common conditions seen in clinical practice are the degenerative joint diseases, including osteoarthrosis (Figures 6.27 and 6.28), and degenerative disorders of the spine. Primary osteoarthrosis causes degeneration of the joint in the absence of any underlying abnormality, whereas secondary osteoarthrosis is related to changes to the joint as a consequence of a pre-existing disorder. Other important conditions affecting joints include rheumatoid arthritis (a polyarticular synovial inflammatory process) (Figure 6.29), juvenile chronic arthritis, ankylosing spondylitis and infectious (septic) arthritis. A detailed discussion of these disorders is beyond the scope of this book, but further information on pathophysiology and radiographic appearances is given in Table 6.7.

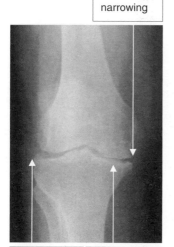

Joint space narrowing

Marginal osteophytes

Subchondral sclerosis

Figure 6.27 An antero-posterior view of the knee joint demonstrating classic osteoarthritic changes.

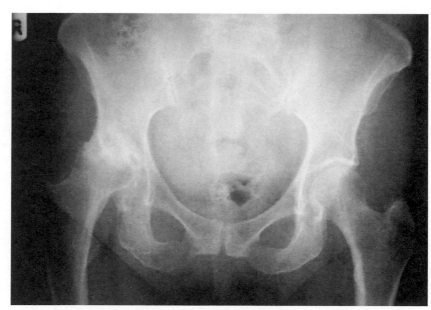

Figure 6.28 Advanced osteoarthritis of the right hip. When compared to the unaffected hip, the diseased joint shows severe narrowing and malalignment, with extensive osteophyte formation. Note also the buttressing (widening) of the neck of femur as a response to abnormal load-bearing stresses.

Six

Table 6.7 Features of a range of joint pathologies.

Type	Region	Features	Radiographic appearances
Primary osteoarthritis (OA)	Hip, knee, foot, hand (DIP and first CMC), AC joint, SI joint, lumbar facets	Mainly females >40 years Idiopathic – no known cause Pain after use, some stiffness in mornings, joint stiffness, crepitus and loss of use Subluxation and deformity when advanced, bony enlargements around joints (e.g. Heberden's or Bouchard's nodes)	May be normal at first Irregular joint space narrowing (loss of cartilage from weight-bearing parts) Subchondral bone sclerosis and cysts Osteophyte formation in non-weight-bearing areas Subluxation and deformity, with possible loose bodies within the joint space No osteoporosis or soft tissue swelling May be abnormal calcifications (e.g. loose bodies, chondrocalcinosis)
Secondary OA	Shoulder, elbow, knee, hip, hand, foot, etc.	Both sexes, > approx. 25 years A predisposing factor is present (e.g. trauma, repetitive stress, metabolic disorder, slipped epiphyses) Clinical findings may be confused by the pre-existing condition	Same as above, but may obscure the presence of the underlying pathology
Inflammatory/erosive OA	Interphalangeal joints of the hand	Females >40 Inflammatory condition Acute, painful swellings of the interphalangeal joints Subluxation and Heberden's nodes	Irregular joint space narrowing Bone erosions Subchondral sclerosis Osteophytes Subluxation
Degenerative conditions of the spine	Particularly lower cervical spine, T2–5, T10–12, and lower lumbar spine All spinal joints may be involved	Both sexes >30 Osteochondrosis affecting discs and subchondral bone Spondylosis, creating osteophytes and bone ridges OA of intervertebral and costovertebral joints Symptoms vary, but include pain and stiffness	Radiographic findings may not correlate well with clinical findings. Findings are very variable Osteophytes and ridging, disc space narrowing, and subchondral bone formation Sclerosis and joint space narrowing

Rheumatoid arthritis (RA)	Hand: MCP and proximal PIP joints, foot, wrist, knee, elbow, shoulder, upper cervical spine, etc.	Females more than males (3:1), 30–60 years approx.
		Chronic multi-system disease, characterised by persistent inflammatory synovitis
		Symmetrical polyarthritis of peripheral joints
		Cartilage destruction, bone erosions, joint deformity
		Pain, tenderness, swelling, morning stiffness, PIP and MCP joints (hands) often involved
		Other abnormalities: rheumatoid nodules under skin, lungs, eyes, cardiac, neurological
			Three stages:
			1 Synovitis
			   soft tissue swelling (fusiform) around affected joints, cortex atrophies, periarticular osteoporosis due to hyperaemia and disuse
			2 Destruction
			   joint space narrowing (cartilage destroyed) marginal and subchondral erosions and cysts
			3 Deformity
			   joint instability, may be fibrous ankylosis gross deformity and subluxation due to ligament abnormalities

Six

Gouty arthritis	Usually big toe	Increased urea level in blood, resulting in uric acid crystallising within joints. Crystals are phagocytosed by leucocytes, which sets up an inflammatory response within the synovium. Extreme pain. Rarely seen in women	Soft tissue swelling only in acute attack. Chronic cases show bone erosions and cysts in periarticular margins. Osteopenia and joint space narrowing. Similar to pseudo gout (chondrocalcinosis), but the latter shows calcification within articular cartilage or menisci
Juvenile chronic arthritis (including Still's disease)	Hips, elbows, knees. Also hand, wrist, cervical spine, other extremities	Both sexes, 5–10 years. Several disorders, including: juvenile onset RA, juvenile onset ankylosing spondylitis, Still's disease. Joint swelling, pain, erythema, with subcutaneous nodules. May be systemic signs	Soft tissue swelling, with osteoporosis around the joint and in the metaphysis. Periostitis and growth disturbances (small, thin bones). Possible joint space loss and erosions in advanced pathology
Ankylosing spondylitis	Axial skeleton; SI joints (site of initial involvement), thoracic + lumbar spine, symphysis pubis, hips, shoulders	Male, 20–30 years. Chronic, progressive inflammatory disease with sacroiliitis as its hallmark. Back and joint pain (particularly SI joint) and stiffness >3 months, with limited movement. Limited chest expansion. Increasing kyphosis. Possible extra-articular findings include uveitis, aortitis, colitis	Spine: marginal syndesmophytes (ossification across intervertebral discs), squaring of vertebrae, disc ossification, anterior ligament ossification (bamboo spine). SI joints: symmetrical bony erosions, fibrosis and ankylosis. Other joints: erosive arthritis similar to RA, osseous ankylosis
Other conditions: psoriatic arthritis, pseudogout, Reiter's syndrome (reactive arthritis)			

DIP, distal interphalangeal (joint); CMC, carpometacarpal (joint); AC, acromioclavicular (joint); SI, sacroiliac (joint); MCP, metacarpophalangeal (joint); PIP, proximal interphalangeal (joint).

Six

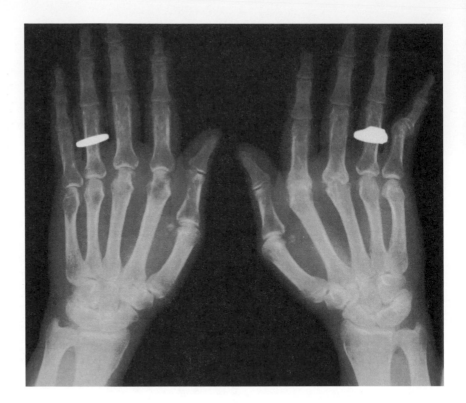

Figure 6.29 Rheumatoid arthritis of both hands. Erosions are noted in the left hand, particularly the head of the third metacarpal. Extensive periarticular osteoporosis is demonstrated. The right hand shows extensive ankylosis and deformity of the second and third metacarpophalangeal joints, and the fifth proximal interphalangeal joint.

Introduction to skeletal injury

The following sections consider the basic mechanics of injury affecting the skeletal system and outline the resulting patterns of trauma in both adult and paediatric patients. Image appearances of trauma and the healing and repair of bone fractures are also discussed.

Mechanisms of injury

Physical injury is typically caused by the transfer of kinetic energy from one body to another, resulting in the production of a wound. Mechanical trauma is related to wound production in four different ways[6]:

(1)   the total amount of energy;
(2)   the duration of the impact;
(3)   the surface area; and
(4)   the tissue characteristics.

For further explanation and examples see Table 6.8. As previously discussed, the tissue characteristics of bone offer both high tensile strength and a degree of elasticity. The high tensile strength of healthy bone requires a very large amount of kinetic energy to result in significant

Six

Table 6.8 Mechanical trauma related to wound production (source: Nowak and Handford[6]).

Characteristic of mechanical trauma	Relation to wound production	Examples
The total amount of energy transferred from one body to another	Using the equation $E = MV^2/2$, where E = kinetic energy, M = mass, V = velocity, one can see that: a heavier object will inflict more damage. In fact doubling the weight of an object will produce twice the energy a faster object will inflict more damage: twice the velocity results in four times the energy	A car which hits a pedestrian will inflict more damage at 60 km/hour than at 30 km/hour. Using the equation for a 50 kg person, the energy imparted by the car would be: At 30 km per hour: $50 \times (30 \times 30)/2 = 22500$ J At 60 km/hour: $50 \times (60 \times 60)/2 = 90000$ J Therefore, four times more energy has been imparted to the pedestrian, resulting in much greater injuries
The duration of the impact	The amount of time over which the energy is imparted. A longer duration impact allows the body tissues to absorb and spread the impact, remaining relatively unharmed	A bullet fired from a gun is travelling at high velocity and has a very short duration of impact, resulting in extensive tissue damage. A bullet tears through tissues and organs, imparting a tremendous amount of energy perpendicular to its path as a result of its rotation
The surface area affected	A larger impact zone allows the kinetic energy to be distributed throughout the tissues, resulting in less serious injury	A horse rider or cyclist who wears a crash helmet is attempting to create a wider impact zone in the event of a fall, allowing the energy to spread outwards within the framework of the helmet, rather than inwards into the skull and brain
The tissue characteristics	Generally tissues with greater elasticity and flexibility will be able to withstand an impact better than tissues which are fixed and rigid Young bones with higher collagen levels are more flexible and less likely to fracture than older, more brittle bones	A jockey whose horse has hit a fence and is falling will react by rolling into a ball (thus protecting his vital organs) and allowing his muscles to relax, as contracted muscles are much more likely to become damaged by the impact. In severe blunt abdominal trauma, the liver is a common site of laceration as it is relatively fixed and rigid. This is even more likely to occur in alcohol abusers whose healthy liver tissue has been replaced by fatty, sclerotic and, therefore, less flexible tissue. Aortic rupture is the most common cause of sudden death in a severe road traffic accident. The aortic arch and thoracic aorta are relatively mobile apart from where they are fixed by a ligament. In the event of a sudden deceleration this ligament attachment holds the arch still whilst the rest of the upper aorta is thrown forward, resulting in a traumatic rupture

Six

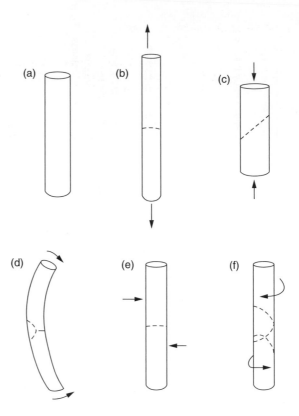

Figure 6.30 Direction of forces (arrows) and the resultant fractures. Remember that usually these forces are often found in combination, complicating the resultant pattern of injury. A long bone is represented by the first cylinder (a). Tension (traction) forces tend to stretch a bone beyond its limits, resulting in a transverse fracture (b). Compression forces often result in an oblique fracture (c). Angulation or bending may cause a transverse fracture with a separate 'butterfly' fragment (d). Shearing forces (two opposing forces) may result in an oblique or transverse fracture with displacement (e). Rotational forces result in a spiral fracture (f).

damage such as a fracture. The elasticity of bone is most evident in children and reduces significantly with advancing age. Ageing bones are much less flexible and more brittle. The patterns of injury as a result of mechanical trauma are therefore likely to differ between different age groups.

The forces imparted to the skeletal system can involve **direct force** (including blunt and penetrating injuries), but the majority of skeletal trauma is as a result of **indirect forces**. Such forces are applied at a distance from the resulting site of injury, which is caused by the transfer of kinetic energy through different tissues until an area of relative weakness is reached. The direction, strength and duration of the applied force provide important clues to help determine the nature of the injury. Figure 6.30 demonstrates the different types of force which may result in fractures, though frequently these forces occur in combination.

Fractures

Fractures may be classified in a number of ways as shown in Table 6.9. When describing a bone fracture within a radiographic report, the following information is important.

Table 6.9   Classifications of fractures.

Severity of fracture	
Open	Fragment of bone protrudes through perforated skin, or presence of an open wound communicating with fracture site. High infection risk
Closed	Skin not perforated
Extent of fracture	
Complete	Bone broken into at least two fragments (e.g. transverse, oblique, spiral)
Incomplete	Fracture does not extend completely across the bone (e.g. greenstick, buckle, torus)
Comminuted	Bone is broken into more than two pieces. High impact/crush injuries. Often take longer to heal as blood supply may be compromised. May include butterfly fracture (wedge-shaped fragment at the apex of the applied force), or segmental fracture (completely separated segment of shaft of a long bone). Butterfly fragment may lack stability
Impacted	One fragment is driven into the cancellous portion of the other fragment (e.g. neck of femur fractures)
Depressed	Fragment driven inwards towards the endosteal side, common in flat bones (e.g. skull) and the tibial plateau
Direction of fracture	
Linear	Fracture line runs parallel to long axis of bone
Transverse	Fracture line runs perpendicular to long axis of bone
Oblique	Fracture line runs obliquely to long axis of bone
Spiral	Fracture line has a helical course around the bone
Dentate	Fracture has rough, toothed broken ends
Stellate	Fracture lines radiating from a central point (e.g. skull fractures)
Other classifications	
Pathological/insufficiency	Fracture through a bone weakened by a disease process (e.g. tumour/infection)
Stress/fatigue fracture	Fracture resulting from repeated loading of bone, with each loading applying less force than that normally expected to fracture a bone. Often caused by athletic or occupational over-use (e.g. metatarsal and tibial fractures in runners, lumbar spondylolysis in manual work)
Chronic stress injury (children)	Repetitive or vigorous activity in child athletes can result in over-loading of the growth plate, which becomes irregular, widened and may have underlying sclerosis of the metaphysis

(a)   (b)   (c)   (d)   (e)   (f)

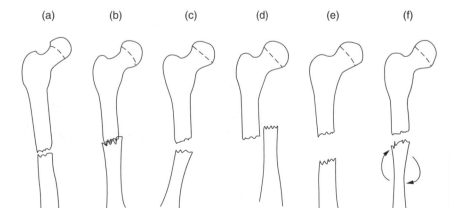

Figure 6.31   Distraction/angulation/displacement. Position of the distal fracture fragment: fracture in normal alignment (a); impacted (b); angulation (c); overlap/bayonet (d); distraction (e); rotational deformity (f).

Six

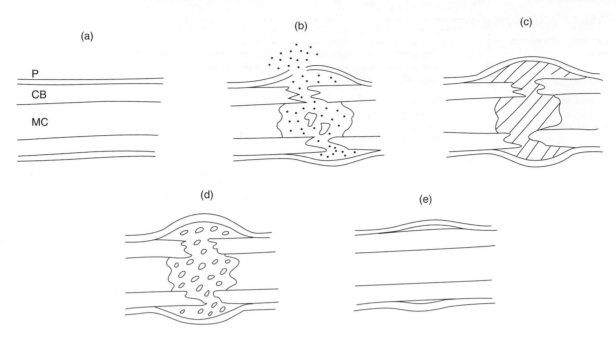

Figure 6.32 Stages of fracture healing: (a) undamaged bone showing a section through compact bone (CB), medullary cavity (MC) and periosteum (P); (b) haematoma builds up with in the medullary cavity after a fracture and strips periosteum away from compact bone: (c) formation of granulation tissue within haematoma; (d) fibrocartilaginous callus formation followed by ossification by hard callus; (e) remodelling.

- **Position** – name and part of fractured bone (e.g. distal third of femur).
- **Type** – of fracture/orientation (e.g. transverse, oblique, spiral).
- **Apposition, alignment** and **rotation** – usually of the distal fragment relative to the proximal fragment (e.g. posterior angulation of the distal fragment). See Figure 6.31.

Apposition refers to the degree of contact between the bone ends, and may be described as anatomical (contacting), or displaced (anterior/posterior, lateral or medial). The degree of displacement may be expressed as a percentage of the cross-sectional diameter of the bone (e.g. 50% displacement). Loss of apposition (distraction) occurs when there is a complete loss of contact between the bone ends, often with soft tissue interposed between the fragments. The overlapping of fragments, where the shafts are in contact, is known as bayonet apposition.

The degree of rotation of the fragments can only be determined correctly if both distal and proximal joints are included on one film. Rotated fragments remodel poorly. Alignment expresses the relation between the long axes of the fracture fragments; its loss is termed angulation. It is identified by the direction of displacement of the distal fragment, which could include varus angulation (distal part of distal fragment points towards the midline of the body) or valgus angulation (distal part points away). When one reads a report there should be sufficient information

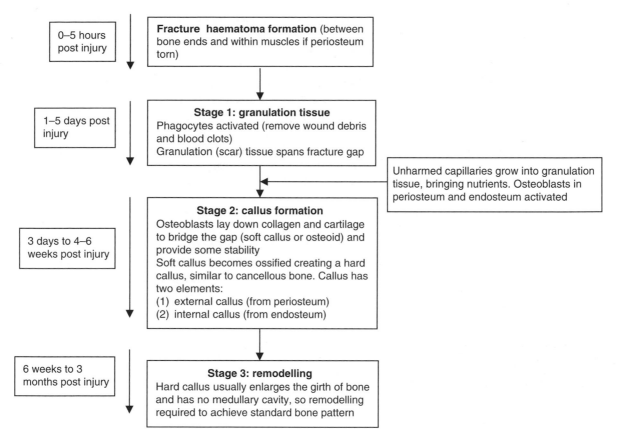

Figure 6.33 The stages of fracture repair.

available to create a mental picture of the fracture in the mind of the reader, even if the actual images are unavailable.

Fracture healing

Although bone has relatively well-developed regenerative powers, healing in connective tissues is generally a prolonged process due to the limited blood supply. The immediate consequence of a bone fracture is the formation of a **haematoma** between the ends of the bone fragments, although blood will also accumulate in the surrounding muscles if the periosteum is torn. Fracture repair begins almost immediately, and there are three stages of healing as shown in Figures 6.32 and 6.33.

- Stage 1 – formation of granulation tissue
- Stage 2 – callus formation
- Stage 3 – remodelling

Uncomplicated fracture repair is so effective that in children little evidence of a previous fracture will remain eight weeks post injury, though

Six

in adults this process takes longer. Some fractures are complicated by confounding factors such as the severity of the initial trauma or underlying pathology.

A pathological fracture caused by an underlying bone disease (such as an infection or a bone tumour) will weaken the bone sufficiently to result in delayed healing. It is essential that the underlying condition is recognised and treated appropriately. Tables 6.4 and 6.5 (pp. 80 and 82, respectively) outline the key radiographic appearances of commonly encountered bone infections and tumours. However, further reading of texts such as *Handbook of Skeletal Radiology*[7] is essential to ensure such conditions are not missed during reporting as this could affect subsequent patient management.

Delayed union is the term used to describe a fracture in which the soft callus is slow to ossify. There are a number of causes of delayed union as outlined in Table 6.10. **Malunion** occurs when a fracture heals in a mis-aligned position (excessive angular or rotational deformity), and is often a temporary phenomenon in children that may disappear with

Table 6.10 Causes of delayed healing.

Factor	Reason why it may result in delayed healing
Avascularity of region	Impaired blood supply will limit the inflow of vital nutrients, oxygen and cells (e.g. osteoblasts). Some regions are particularly susceptible to vascular problems, including the hip and scaphoid
Advancing age	The elderly generally have impaired blood flow, reduced dietary intake and metabolism and may have underlying bone disorders (e.g. osteoporosis)
Metabolic disorders	Hormonal problems (e.g. hyperparathyroidism) may interfere with the metabolism of calcium or other vital constituents of bone
Inadequate initial reduction	A large physical distance (more than 2 cm) between the bone ends will cause difficulties for the granulation tissue and callus to bridge the gap. Anteroposterior angulation may remodel well, but lateral (varus/valgus) angulation remodels poorly. Rotational deformities do not remodel effectively[7]
Inadequate immobilisation	Too much movement at the fracture site will dislodge the vulnerable granulation tissue, and will tear immature blood vessels
Pathological fractures	The presence of underlying bone disease will make fracture repair slow or even impossible. Tumours will disrupt the normal function of osteoblasts and osteoclasts, and metabolic bone disease such as osteoporosis will weaken the bone framework across which the fracture must be bridged
Infection	The presence of pathogens will stimulate an inflammatory response, interfering with normal healing
Diet inadequate	A diet deficient in vital nutrients (e.g. calcium, vitamin D and C), or the body's ability to metabolise correctly will interfere with fracture repair
Comminuted fractures	A complex fracture involves a number of fracture repair zones. The presence of small, necrosed or dead fragments will impair blood supply and set up infection sites
Foreign bodies	Presence of foreign bodies may introduce infection and movement across the fracture repair site
Surgical fixation	Internal fixation of fractures will limit minor movements of the fracture ends. Such movements help to stimulate bone growth. External fixation devices can be used to regularly manipulate the fracture ends, thus stimulating growth Surgery will also disperse the haematoma, which is important as a structure in which granulation tissue can build

Six

further skeletal growth. **Non-union** describes a fracture which is still not completely united after six to nine months. A non-united bone is often characterised by an associated **pseudoarthrosis**, or false joint, which is created at the fracture site by persistent movement between the bone ends. Such problems occur in bones that are insufficiently immobilised, particularly in the scaphoid, femoral neck, tibia, clavicle and the odontoid peg[8]. They may be relatively painless, but do not permit adequate weight bearing.

Fractures in children

Children can experience any of the fractures described in Table 6.9 (p. 93), but there are also a number of trauma patterns specifically associated with the immature skeleton. The increased porosity of immature bones results in a higher incidence of incomplete fractures, including the following.

- The **greenstick** fracture is a break through only one cortex extending into the medullary cavity, but the opposite cortex is usually unaffected (although it can be affected by angulation or bulging). It is caused by tension to the cortex, and commonly affects the distal third of the radius and ulna.
- The **torus** fracture is caused by a compressive force which buckles but does not break the cortex, often seen in the distal radius and ulna.
- The **lead pipe** fracture is a combination of greenstick in one bone and torus fractures in the adjacent (or same) bone.
- The **bowing** (or plastic bowing) fracture is commonly seen in the forearm and fibula and is a response to longitudinal stress. It usually occurs in the 2–5 year age group, where the bones are particularly pliable, allowing bending rather than breaking of the cortex. These fractures are often subtle and difficult to detect but may be accompanied by a greenstick fracture of the adjacent bone.

The so-called 'toddler's fracture' is found in children between one and three years of age. It is usually an undisplaced, oblique fracture of the long bones (usually the distal tibia, fibula or femur). Such fractures may be difficult to detect radiographically, especially in the absence of a clear clinical history.

Growth plate injuries

Up to 15% of all long bone fractures in children under 16 years of age involve the growth plate. The majority of such injuries are found in the distal radius (50%), distal humerus (17%) and distal tibia and fibula (20%)[8]. Growth plate injuries have serious implications as there is a high potential for growth deformity at the site of the injury. They are

Six

Type	Description	Diagrammatic representation
SH I (6%)	Fracture through the growth plate, possibly resulting in the epiphysis slipping out of line with the diaphysis, e.g. slipped epiphyses of the femoral head	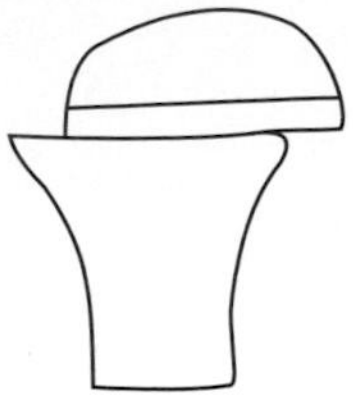
SH II (75%)	Fracture through part of the growth plate which extends into the metaphysis. A triangular wedge of the metaphysis may be attached to the plate (metaphyseal 'corner' sign). Prognosis for healing without deformity is good	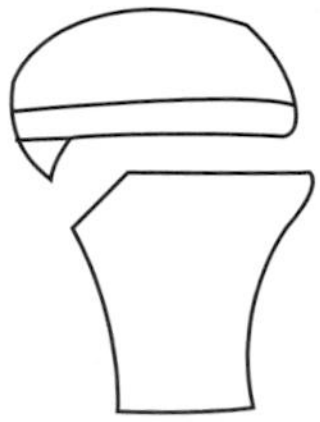
SH III (8%)	A fracture through part of the growth plate, extending into the epiphysis (usually a vertical fracture). Any fracture involving the epiphysis has the potential to damage the dividing cells in the proliferative zone of the growth plate, thus leading to possible growth disturbance	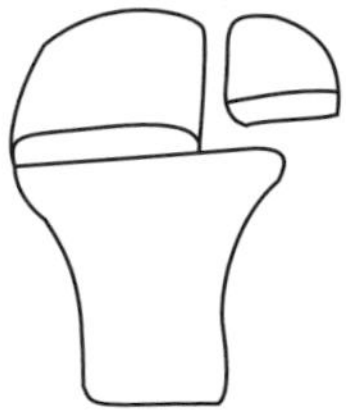
SH IV (10%)	A vertical fracture extending from the articular cartilage, through the epiphysis and growth plate, and into the metaphysis. See SH III notes above	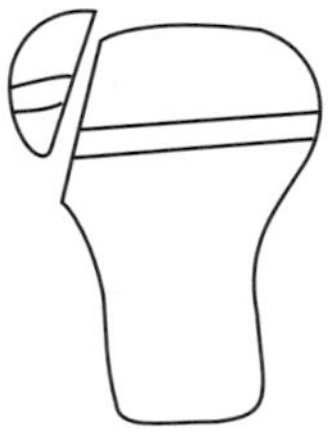
SH V (1%)	Crushing or compressing of the epiphyseal plate. There may be no obvious fracture or angulation of bone, thus resulting in a potential for false negative results, or mis-diagnosis as an SH I. Very high complication rates, with partial premature closure of the growth plate and resultant major growth disturbance/deformity	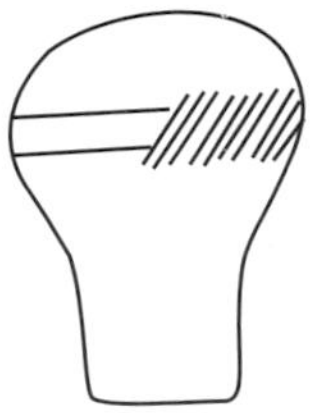

Figure 6.34   The Salter–Harris (SH) classification of growth plate injuries.

described following the **Salter–Harris classification,** graded from I to V in order of ascending severity (Figure 6.34). Salter–Harris V is of particular concern, as the injury results in complete crushing of a section of the growth plate. The absence of an osseous fracture means that this injury is frequently overlooked. A retrospective diagnosis may be made

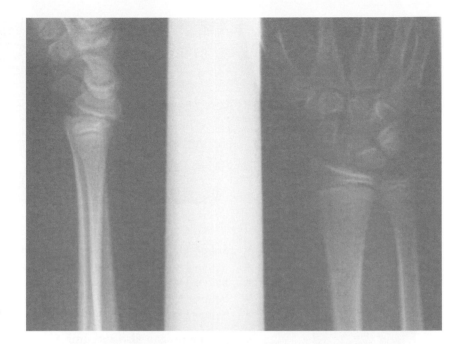

Figure 6.35 Salter–Harris 1 of the distal radius. The fracture has traversed the growth plate and caused the epiphysis to slip posteriorly. The fracture is difficult to identify on the postero-anterior view.

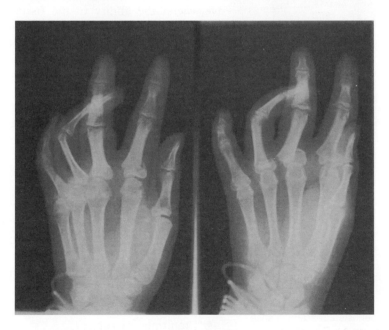

Figure 6.36 Severe trauma has resulted in Salter–Harris (SH) fractures involving the second to fifth proximal phalanges. The fourth proximal phalanx is a displaced SH I, but the others are mainly SH IIs. Note the metaphyseal fractures on the second and fifth fingers.

when a further radiograph reveals early fusion of the growth plate. Salter–Harris I injuries can also be subtle, although the presence of suspicious soft tissue changes (e.g. elevation of wrist pronator fat pad, or soft tissue swelling in the ankle) should raise the possibility of a growth plate injury (Figures 6.35 and 6.36). An easy way to memorise the above classification and related injury patterns is given below.

Six

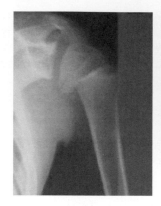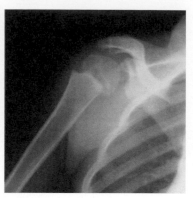

Figure 6.37 Slipped upper humeral epiphyses. Rapid growth introduces greater shearing forces on a weakened growth plate. The epiphysis is shortened and the growth plate widened.

- Salter–Harris I –   **S**lipped epiphysis
- Salter–Harris II – **A**bove epiphysis
- Salter–Harris III – **L**ower than epiphysis
- Salter–Harris IV – **T**hrough the epiphysis
- Salter–Harris V – **R**ammed epiphysis

Growth plates can also succumb to **repetitive stress injury**, which can overwhelm the ability of the tissue to cope. Such stress injuries are common in child athletes such as gymnasts, resulting in widened growth plates with accompanying sclerosis of the metaphysis. Similarly, relatively minor trauma can precipitate injury to a growth plate already weakened by particularly rapid growth. This may result in a slipped epiphysis (similar to a Salter–Harris I), usually of the femoral capital epiphysis, known as a SUFE (slipped upper femoral epiphysis). Over time the epiphyseal plate appears to widen, and the epiphysis itself shortens. Occasionally other rapidly growing bones can be affected, including the proximal humerus (Figure 6.37).

Non-accidental injury

Non-accidental injury (NAI) in children is a distressing issue for all concerned, and is estimated to affect approximately 10% of all children seen in a trauma department[8]. There are a number of radiographic findings which raise the suspicion of physical child abuse, particularly in those under four years old:

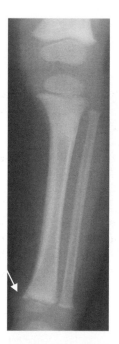

Figure 6.38 The radiographic signs of non-accidental injury (NAI) can be very subtle. A faint periosteal reaction is seen on the medial tibial border, accompanied by a medial metaphyseal corner fracture (arrow) of the tibia. Also known as a classic metaphyseal lesion, it is virtually pathognomic for NAI. The injuries are often bilateral, as in this case.

- multiple fractures;
- unusual fractures (e.g. scapula, rib fractures). Rib fractures under two years of age are usually caused by severe squeezing;
- fractures in different stages of healing (much abuse is repetitive);
- any long bone fractures in children under 12 months, particularly humeral fractures in infants and femoral fractures in crawling children (i.e. before children are fully mobile and able to inflict serious damage on themselves);

- subperiosteal haemorrhage with periostitis – a raised periosteum;
- metaphyseal corner fractures, or classic metaphyseal lesions (CML), often seen in children under 18 months (Figure 6.38);
- transverse diaphyseal or metaphyseal fractures (caused by a traction force, such as pulling an extremity);
- the fracture is not compatible with the given clinical history or where the history is absent.

One should remember, however, that there are a number of potential differential diagnoses for most of the above findings, including pure accidental injury, normal growth changes of the metaphysis and periosteum, and diseases such as **osteogenesis imperfecta**. However, one should note that a diagnosis of CML is virtually pathognomic for NAI, and is caused by the rapid acceleration and deceleration of flailing limbs when an infant is shaken. Appropriate NAI protocols should always be followed if suspicion is raised by the radiographic findings.

Injuries to soft tissues and joints

A force sufficient to fracture normal bone will inevitably affect the soft tissues, but significant soft tissue damage can be found in the absence of bone injury, making diagnosis of soft tissue injury more problematic (see Salter–Harris V above). Plain films will not always demonstrate the degree of damage sufficiently, as tissues often recoil back to their original position. Alternative imaging modalities (in particular magnetic resonance imaging and ultrasound) may be indicated to assess the integrity of soft tissues in and around a joint.

Following a bone fracture, the potential for **secondary injury** is high. Fragments of bone can move against vessels and organs resulting in lacerations and contusions. In particular rib, pelvis and skull fragments can contribute to damage of the underlying organs. The initial force applied to the body can also cause primary damage to the soft tissues, which all respond differently to trauma.

Ligaments

Ligaments are made of dense fibrous connective tissue and serve to stabilise and strengthen joints. If excessive force is applied to a particular joint the ligaments will tear. A **partial tear** (grade 2 moderate sprain) leaves some of the ligament intact, giving some degree of stability, but a **complete tear** (grade 3 rupture) will lead to a highly unstable joint. If the force was great enough to separate the bones, but they then return to their original position, the joint is **sprained**. If the bones of the joint remain totally displaced, the joint is **dislocated** or **luxated**. A partial loss of contact between two articulating bones is called a **subluxation**. Some degree of joint capsule and ligament tearing and bleeding will always be

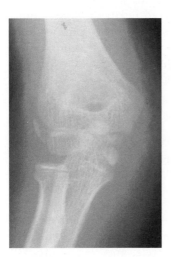

Figure 6.39 An avulsion fracture of the medial epicondyle is seen as a clearly defined flake of bone.

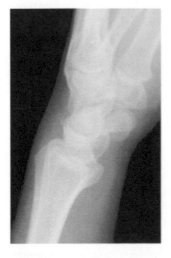

Figure 6.40 A flake of bone is seen on the dorsal aspect of the carpal bones. It is most probably an avulsion fracture of the triquetral bone.

Six

associated with a dislocation. If the damaged ligament lies within the joint capsule (such as the cruciate ligaments of the knee) blood will mix with the synovial fluid and delay healing. Some ligamentous injuries are particularly complex. In the knee joint, for example, the medial collateral ligament is attached firmly to the medial meniscus, an incomplete ring of fibrocartilage within the joint space. Twisting injuries to the knee can result in the ligament tearing the meniscus to which it is attached, leaving a challenging injury to repair. Ruptured ligaments may require surgery to create good apposition, but a partial tear often requires only conservative management. The absence of a good blood supply results in a long recovery period of up to six months.

Tendons

Tendons transmit the contractile forces of muscle to bone, and both compressive and severe stretching forces can cause a tear. Ageing tendons are more susceptible to injury and require a longer period of healing. Scar tissue formation is often found to interfere with future function. Occasionally a tendon or ligament under sudden strain can pull off a fragment from the underlying bone – this is known as an **avulsion fracture** (Figures 6.39 and 6.40). Such injuries are commonly seen in large tendon insertions including the olecranon, tibial tubercle, and several areas of the pelvis and hip.

Muscles

Muscles can also suffer damage due to high contractile loads, excessive stretching forces or compression (such as a direct blow). Tearing of a muscle will usually be accompanied by bleeding which can be severe in muscles which are exercising at the time of the injury. These muscle haematomas may lead to scar formation or **myositis ossificans** in large muscle groups. This condition is characterised by a well-defined region of intramuscular ossification parallel to the long axis of the bone, seen usually six to eight weeks post injury (Figure 6.41).

Cartilage

Cartilage injury within a joint can be accompanied by underlying bone injury (osteochondral fracture) or can be seen in the absence of bone injury (chondral fracture), following dislocations or subluxations. It is usually found in conjunction with painful joint effusions, joint locking and limitation of motion. The cartilage heals by fibrous repair, whereby scar tissue is created by the perichondrium covering the cartilage surface. Any cartilage fragments are usually reabsorbed, but some loss of joint function can occur. In adolescents with joint symptoms a diagnosis of **osteochondritis dissecans** (OCD) must be considered, particularly if asso-

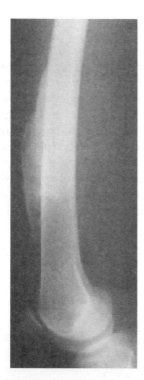

Figure 6.41   A lateral view of the femur demonstrating post-traumatic ossification within muscle, known as myositis ossificans. The differential diagnosis is osteosarcoma, so careful diagnostic work-up is necessary.

Six

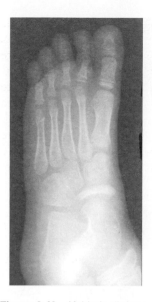

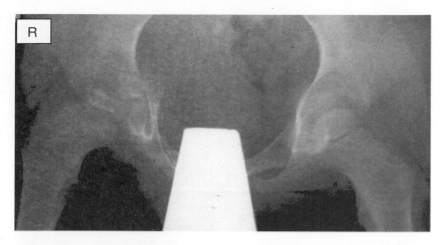

Figure 6.42 Legg–Calvé–Perthes disease (osteochondrosis of the femoral head). Bone necrosis has led to fragmentation and shortening of the right femoral head. Growth abnormalities within the metaphysis lead to cyst formation and a short, wide neck (compare with the left side).

Figure 6.43 Kohler's disease (osteochondrosis) of the navicular bone. Reactive sclerosis is evidence of bone necrosis, though in the absence of pain a normal variant of ossification should be considered.

ciated with the medial femoral condyle or talus. OCD may or may not follow significant trauma and results in a portion of the articular surface fragmenting. Adolescents and children are also susceptible to similar conditions affecting subarticular bone, known collectively as **osteochondroses**. These problems may result in patchy osteonecrosis, characterised by reactive bone sclerosis and cysts, subchondral collapse and potential joint space narrowing. They are caused by trauma or excessive stress loads, though sometimes the causative factors are not identified. One should be cautious, however, as many normal variants have fragmented ossification centres which simulate the osteochondroses. Examples of the latter include:

- **Osgood–Schlatter's disease** of the tibial tubercle (11–15 year olds);
- **Perthes' disease** of the femoral head epiphysis (4–8 year olds) (Figure 6.42);
- **Kohler's disease** of the navicular bone (3–6 year olds) (Figure 6.43);
- **Sinding–Larsen–Johanssen disease** of the patella (11–15 year olds) (Figure 6.44);
- **Kienbock's disease** of the lunate bone (20–40 year olds).

Radiographic signs of joint injury may include the presence of a dislocation or subluxation, avulsion fractures, joint effusions and fluid levels. A **joint effusion** usually occurs several hours after injury, and is characterised by an excess of synovial fluid. Rapidly accumulating joint effusion is normally the result of bleeding from a torn ligament and is known as a **haemarthrosis**. A **lipohaemarthrosis** contains both blood and lipid collections within the joint, seen as a fluid–fluid level on a horizontal beam radiograph (Figures 6.45 and 6.46). The lipids seep out of the fatty yellow marrow within the bone epiphyses and are therefore a strong indi-

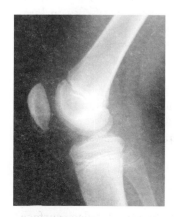

Figure 6.44 Osteochondrosis of the patella. Note the fragmented and avulsed inferior pole.

Six

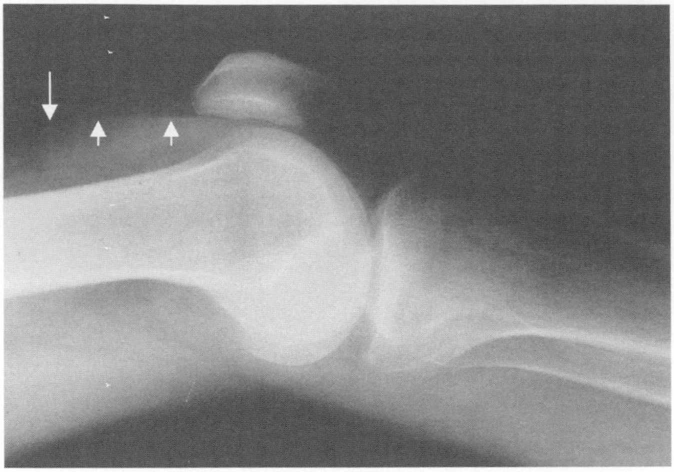

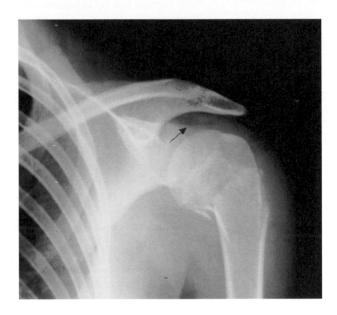

Figure 6.45
Lipohaemarthrosis in the knee. Horizontal beam lateral knee projection demonstrates a lipohaemarthrosis, seen as a fat–blood fluid level adjacent to the posterior border of the patella (arrow).

Figure 6.46
Lipohaemarthrosis in the shoulder. An obvious comminuted fracture of the proximal humerus. Note also the lipohaemarthrosis within the joint cavity (arrow).

cation of an intra-articular fracture. When air is seen within the joint as an air–fluid interface (**pneumolipohaemarthrosis**), severe trauma such as a fracture dislocation or open fracture is normally suspected.

References

1 Gray, H. (1980). In: Warwick, R. and Williams, P.L. (eds.) *Gray's Anatomy*, 36th edn. Churchill Livingstone, Edinburgh.

Six

2   Gunn, C. (2002) *Bones and Joints: A Guide for Students*, 4th edn. Churchill Livingstone, Edinburgh.
3   Calder, C. and Chessel, G. (1988) *An Atlas of Radiological Interpretation: The Bones.* Wolfe Medical Publications Ltd, London.
4   Greulich, W.W. and Pyle, S.I. (1959) *Radiographic Atlas of Skeletal Development of the Hand and Wrist*, 2nd edn. Stanford University Press, Stanford.
5   Keats, T.E. and Smith, S. (1988) *An Atlas of Normal Developmental Roentgen Anatomy*, Year Book Medical Publishers, Chicago.
6   Nowak, T.J. and Handford, A.G. (1999) *Essentials of Pathophysiology: Concepts and Applications for the Health Care Professions*, 2nd edn. McGraw-Hill, Boston.
7   Manaster, B.J. (1997) *Handbook of Skeletal Radiology*, 2nd edn. Mosby-Year Book Inc, St Louis.
8   Taylor, J. and Resnick, D. (2000) *Skeletal Imaging Atlas of the Spine and the Extremities.* W.B. Saunders, Philadelphia.

Further reading

Adler, C.P. (2000) *Bone Diseases: Macroscopic, Histological, and Radiological Diagnosis of Structural Changes in the Skeleton.* Springer-Verlag, Berlin.
Gunn, C. (2002) *Bones and Joints: A Guide for Students*, 4th edn. Churchill Livingstone, Edinburgh.
Keats, T.E. (1996) *Atlas of Normal Roentgen Variants that May Simulate Disease*, 6th edn. Year Book Medical Publishers, Chicago.
Kohler, A. and Zimmer, E.A. (1993) *Borderlands of Normal and Early Pathologic Findings in Skeletal Radiography*, 4th edn. Thieme Medical Publishers, New York.
Resnick, D. and Niwayama, G. (1994) *Diagnosis of Bone and Joint Disorders*, 3rd edn. W.B. Saunders, Philadelphia.
Taylor, J. and Resnick, D. (2000) *Skeletal Imaging Atlas of the Spine and the Extremities.* W.B. Saunders, Philadelphia.

Six

Section Two

Section Two

7 Skeletal Trauma of the Upper Limb

Jonathan McConnell

Introduction

This chapter will look at the radiographic appearances seen in trauma to the upper limb. The major patterns and mechanisms will be discussed, starting at the fingers. In each section the differences in appearances seen in paediatric skeletal images will also be described.

General considerations

Despite appearing to be fairly innocuous injuries, trauma to the digits can lead to functional impairments that may be disabling for life if not detected. Similarly, injuries to the carpal bones or the joints of the carpus can be equally incapacitating.

The common fall on the outstretched hand (FOOSH) may produce a range of different injury appearances that are closely linked to age and skeletal maturity[1]. Variations in the way that falls occur, and in the forces involved, generate specific and pathognomic image patterns.

It is prudent to consider the forearm as a ring structure so that it may be assessed according to patterns typically seen within 'circular' arrangements. Injuries to these bones often result from a FOOSH incident, and where fracture does not occur in both bones, a strong association with joint dislocation or ligament injury has been seen. Imaginary lines have been devised to assist in review of the elbow – acronyms such as CRITOL (see p. 146) have been suggested for reliable scrutiny of the secondary ossification centres of the juvenile joint. Associated patterns of soft tissue injury may also be seen in the plain film. The shoulder and proximal humerus also display different injury patterns at various stages of life.

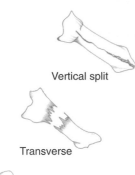

Vertical split

Transverse

Comminuted

Figure 7.1   Phalangeal fractures.

Each area of the upper limb has special radiographic projections associated with it. The need for good standard projections cannot be overemphasised; however, at times, further projections may be necessary to confirm clinical suspicions. The shoulder joint, owing to its complexity, probably has the largest number of radiographic examinations, each tailored to elucidate specific injuries[2].

The hand

Avulsion injuries, particularly of the fingers, are easily missed and are functionally important.

The fingers

Most injuries to the fingers occur by crushing, twisting and avulsive forces (hyperextension/flexion)[3].

Phalangeal fractures (Figure 7.1)

- Fracture to the tufts (distal ends) (Figure 7.2).
- Shaft fracture – usually angulated, the degree of which is underestimated unless visualised on the lateral film.
- Avulsion fracture of the phalangeal dorsal or volar corners at the sites of ligamentous insertions.

Several important injuries occur in the fingers. These are demonstrated in Figure 7.3.

- **Mallet deformity** – results from either a tendon injury or a dorsal intra-articular avulsion fracture at the base of the distal phalanx (Figure 7.4).
- **Boutonniere deformity** – proximal interphalangeal (PIP) flexion with distal interphalangeal (DIP) extension and rupture of the middle slip (band) of the extensor mechanism as it passes over the flexed PIP. The DIP is pulled effectively into hyperextension so the PIP 'button holes' the middle slip. Avulsion of the dorsum of the base of the middle phalanx may occur.

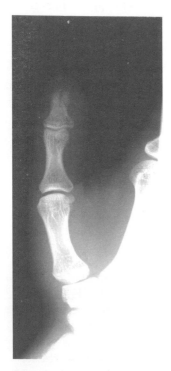

Figure 7.2   Radiograph showing vertical splitting fracture of the distal phalanx of the right thumb.

Self-test answer

A comminuted, vertical splitting fracture is evidenced by the lucent line seen in the distal phalanx of the right thumb.

(a)

Boutonniere deformity

(b)

Phalangeal base fracture

(c)

Fracture of phalangeal base
at extensor tendon insertion

Mallet deformity

(d)

Volar plate insertion avulsion

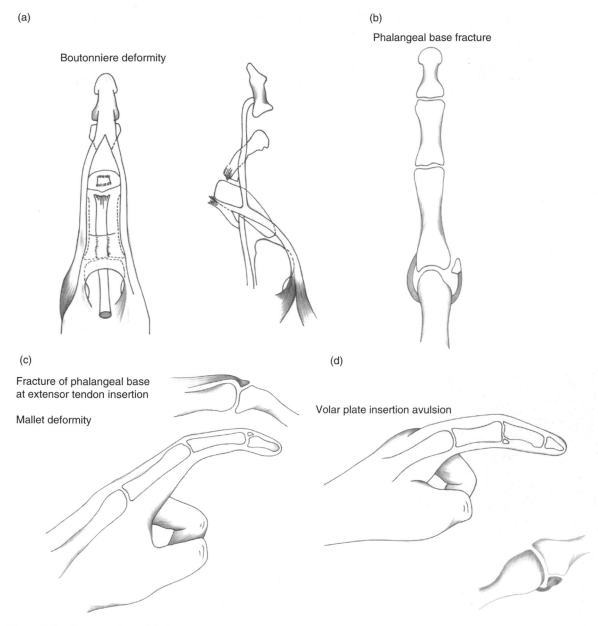

Figure 7.3 Common finger injuries.

- **Avulsion of a volar fragment** – forced hyperextension of a flexed finger avulses the flexor digitorum profundis from the volar aspect to produce either a pure tendon injury or an intra-articular avulsion fracture.
- **Volar plate fracture** – crossing the MCP (metacarpophalangeal)

Seven

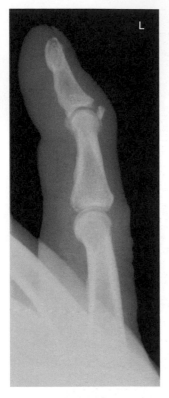

L

Figure 7.4   Mallet deformity of the left index finger.

and PIP joints, the volar plate has a weak proximal attachment but stronger distal attachment to the volar aspect of the base of the middle phalanx. On hyperextension this distal attachment will avulse, producing a fragment from the volar side of the base of the middle phalanx. This may also be seen in conjunction with a mallet finger.

- **Collateral ligament injury** – found at all MCP, PIP and DIP joints, the most common injury is avulsion of the ulnar collateral ligament of the proximal phalanx of the thumb – 'gamekeeper's thumb' – due to valgus (thumb bent away from the midline) injury.

Phalangeal dislocations

Forced hyperextension of the thumb or finger joints is the usual cause for these injuries. Normally the distal segment is displaced posteriorly (Figure 7.5) relative to the proximal portion. Take care to scrutinise the bones carefully for any associated avulsion injuries that might be hidden by the spectacular appearance of the dislocated segment. Oblique projections may be helpful[4].

The metacarpals

Injuries occur primarily in the fifth metacarpal with the first metacarpal closely following in frequency. Other metacarpal injuries (singly or multiply) are often the result of a badly timed impact, for example a mistimed punch or fall on a clenched fist[5].

Fractures of the first metacarpal

- 78% involve the proximal portion of the bone.
- 10% involve the shaft.
- 12% involve the neck and head.

Eponymous injuries seen in the first metacarpal are as follows (Figures 7.6–7.8).

Self-test answer

A rounded piece of bone is seen inferior to the distal phalanx of the left index finger. There is an apparent jig-saw fit of this portion of bone with the postero-inferior corner of the distal phalanx typical of the appearances seen in a mallet finger.

Seven

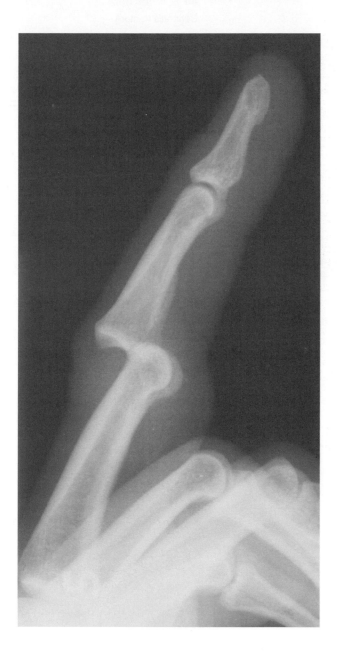

Figure 7.5 Posterior dislocation of the middle phalanx of the right middle finger.

Self-test answer

Through moving postero-inferiorly the middle phalanx of the right middle finger has lost its alignment with the apical articular surface of the proximal phalanx commensurate with a posterior dislocation.

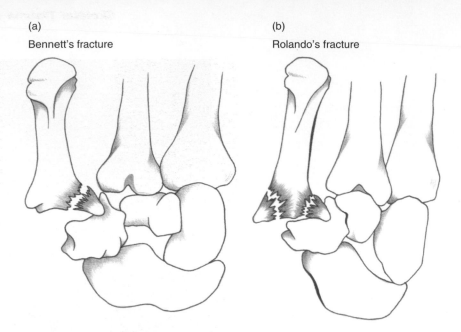

(a)
Bennett's fracture

(b)
Rolando's fracture

Figure 7.6 (a, b) Intra-articular first metacarpal base fractures.

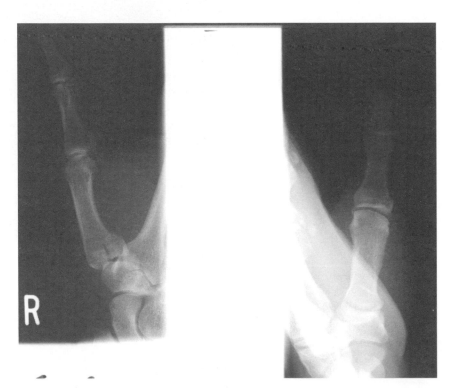

Figure 7.7 Right thumb showing Bennett's fracture.

Self-test answer

A vertical lucent line is seen intersecting the proximal articular surface of the first metacarpal resulting in the separation of a portion of bone on the ulnar aspect. This appearance is consistent with a Bennett's fracture of the right thumb.

Seven

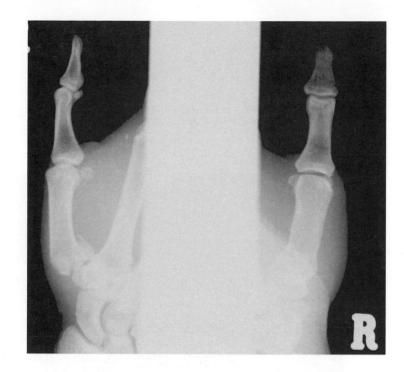

Figure 7.8   Right thumb displaying a Rolando-type intra-articular fracture.

- **Bennett's fracture** – which displays dorsal subluxation or dislocation of the metacarpal with a fracture involving the volar lip of the metacarpal.
- **Rolando's fracture** – has a T- or Y-shaped articular surface comminuted component.

Extra-articular fractures

It is important to assess whether an oblique fracture enters the joint as most extra-articular fractures can be treated by closed means. The range of metacarpal base fractures is shown in Figure 7.9.

Other metacarpals (Figures 7.10 and 7.11)

The fractures most frequently seen in the remaining metacarpals are transverse and oblique fractures, which may display angulation or be

Self-test answer

A three-piece fracture is seen in the base of the right first metacarpal. There is some loss of continuity of the usual bony arrangement suggesting subluxation of the ulnar portion of this complex fracture. Appearances are typical of the Rolando type of injury.

Seven

Figure 7.9   The range and position of first metacarpal base fractures.

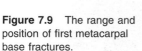

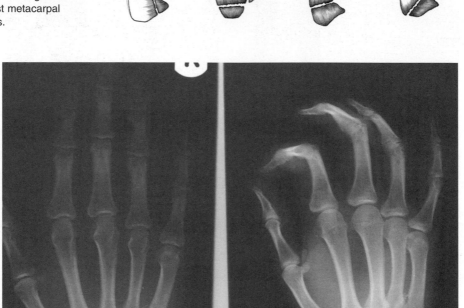

Figure 7.10   Fracture of the bases of the fourth and fifth metacarpals of the right hand.

prone to movement prior to complete healing. Many centres employ lateral films for assessing degree of displacement, and following up conservative treatment of fifth and fourth metacarpal fractures. Other than suspected cases of instability that becomes evident within the first week following injury, this practice has little to add to the management[6].

Self-test answer

There is a loss of cortical integrity and continuity of the base of the right fifth metacarpal. Multiple fragments present are indicative of a comminuted fracture of the base of the fifth metacarpal.

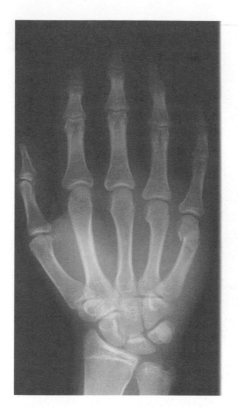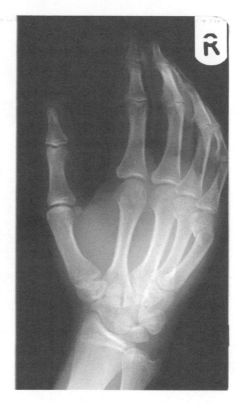

Figure 7.11 Boxer's fracture of the right fifth metacarpal.

The boxer's fracture typically produces a break of the fifth metacarpal neck with a palmar angulation of the metacarpal head, typical of a misdirected punch. The impact of teeth on bone following the assault may lead to subtle intra-articular or bony damage to the third metacarpal head with subsequent development of sepsis[7]. A tangential projection will help elucidate this injury. Osteomyelitis of the injured bone is a serious complication that may be noted with this injury pattern.

More than one metacarpal injury?
Where more than one metacarpal is injured (Figure 7.12) it is often prudent to follow the line of injury generated by fractures in the bones. In this way, evidence of further injury may be spotted at points remote from the obvious abnormality, and associated dislocations of the

Self-test answer

A fracture in the neck of the fifth metacarpal is seen with palmar angulation of the distal portion indicative of the boxer's-type fracture.

Seven

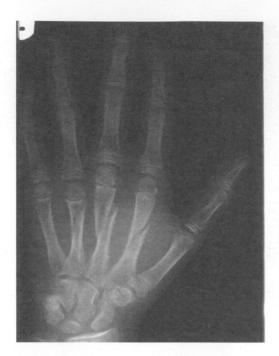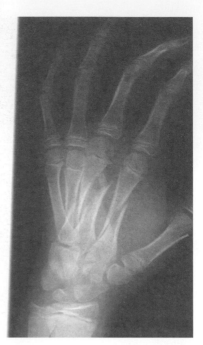

Figure 7.12   Multiple metacarpal fractures in a child.

metacarpal bases are identified. Where the appearances are unclear, the use of a 'ball catcher's' (AP oblique or Norgaard)-type projection may help in diagnosis[8]. Box 7.1 presents a summary of fractures and dislocations seen in children (p. 120). See also Figure 7.13.

Carpometacarpal dislocation

Carpometacarpal (CMC) dislocation (Figures 7.14 and 7.15) is usually assessed on the dorsi-palmar projection by evaluation of the evenly spaced zigzag line of the joint space between the metacarpal and the carpal bones. Although quite rare, the frequency of such injuries is as follows:

- 50% involve the fifth metacarpal;
- 25% involve the second metacarpal;

Self-test answer

Oblique fractures of the left second, third and fourth metacarpals are seen consistent with a trapping/crushing injury of the hand. Minimal displacement is seen; however, a lateral hand projection would allow full evaluation.

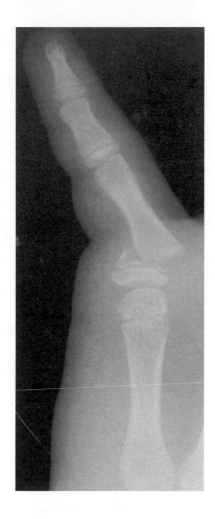

Figure 7.13 At first glance a Salter–Harris II injury – but closer inspection reveals otherwise.

- 80% are multiple and are formed of the fifth metacarpal plus another;
- 66% dislocate dorsally.

Flexion of the fingers may give an appearance of overlap at the CMC joints and hence falsely raise suspicions of injury. Undiagnosed CMC dislocations can result in serious loss of hand function.

Self-test answer

First look at this injury suggests a Salter–Harris type II injury. Closer scrutiny reveals that the fracture line is travelling purely through the metaphyseal region of the bone without involvement of the growth plate.

Box 7.1   Fractures and dislocations of the phalanges and metacarpals in children.

- 50% – proximal phalanx fractures
- 25% – middle phalanx fractures
- 25% – distal phalanx fractures

Phalangeal fractures involve the:

- epiphysis and metaphysis in 41%
- diaphysis in 26%
- intra-articular region in 18%
- and neck of phalanx in 15%

Greenstick and torus fractures are common, particularly at the base of the proximal phalanges and metacarpals. Most epiphyseal injuries are Salter–Harris I or II, a small number are Salter–Harris type III, and less commonly Salter–Harris IV. Type V make up about 1% of injuries.

Salter–Harris type I

- More common in younger children
- Injuries involving the distal phalanx are often associated with significant lacerations of the nail bed
- Osteomyelitis has been reported as a complication of such injuries

Salter–Harris type II

- Demonstrates a small flake or triangular fragment of the metaphysis
- Particularly common at the base of the proximal phalanx

Salter–Harris type III

- Intra-articular and usually occurs at the site of ligamentous or capsular insertion
- The volar portion of the epiphysis of the distal phalanx closes before the dorsal portion. Because of this a Salter–Harris III epiphyseal separation may occur in the distal phalanx of adolescents, which is similar to the baseball finger in adults

Salter–Harris type IV

- Also intra-articular and looks like a combination of types II and III
- Being separated from the main portion of the bone, these injuries are susceptible to slippage and hence early physeal fusion. Often fixation is required to assure a good reduction

Salter–Harris type V

- These injuries have the worst prognosis as they result from physeal crushing with concomitant cessation of bone growth
- Care is required not to misinterpret appearances as growth plate fusion when the injured skeleton is not yet fully mature and there is an underlying serious injury. This is particularly problematic when fusion or injury only includes part of the physeal line

Crushing injuries frequently cause comminution, soft tissue damage and ligamentous tears. As a result of the muscle insertions to the metacarpals and phalanges, fractures regularly mis-align, making reduction more difficult. Punch injuries are frequently encountered in boys as they reach puberty often with palmar angulation of metacarpal neck fractures.

(a)   (b)

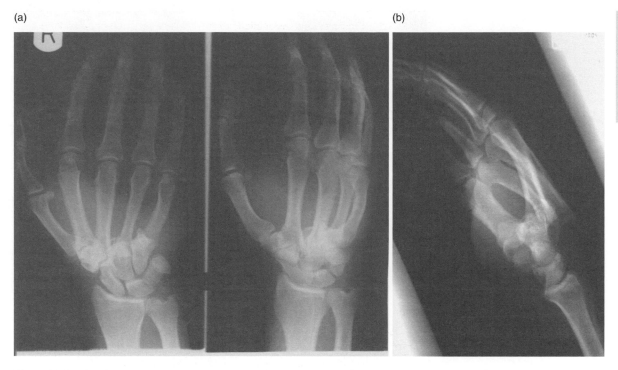

Figure 7.14 (a, b) Dorsi-palmar, oblique and lateral projections showing dislocated second to fifth metacarpals.

The carpus

The carpal bones are a group of eight bones arranged in two rows between the distal radius and ulna and the metacarpal bases. This complex arrangement can be radiographically confusing; although, there are some basic rules of evaluation. The carpus normally demonstrates equal spacing of approximately 2 mm between each bone on the PA radiograph. The normally positioned lunate is trapezoidal but appears triangular following dislocation. It should be remembered that this may present as an artefact in the PA projection if the hand is held in flexion or extension. The lateral projection is used as a baseline for describing the relationship between the radius, lunate, capitate and third metacarpal

Self-test answer

The usual alignment of the CMC joint is lost between the bases of the second to fifth metacarpals as noted by dorsal protuberance of the proximal ends of these bones on the lateral projection. Dislocation of the concomitant CMC joints is apparent. There is no obvious indication of a fracture; however, gross disruption of the soft tissue structures should be inferred.

Seven

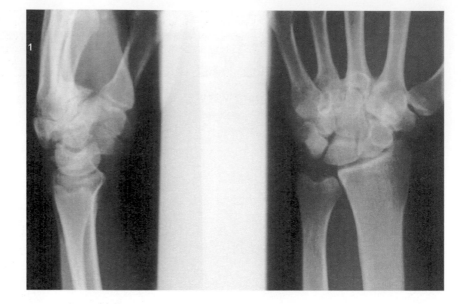

Figure 7.15   PA and lateral wrist projections displaying carpometacarpal joint dislocation.

Lateral wrist carpal alignment

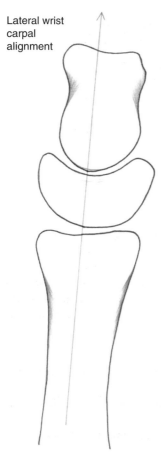

Figure 7.16   Normal lateral wrist relationships.

base with the scaphoid arching out onto the palmar side of the wrist[9]. Figure 7.16 shows the normal lateral wrist relationships.

In the dominant injury scenario (FOOSH), compressive and tensile forces travel through the wrist from the radiocarpal joint, across the proximal and distal carpal rows to the CMC joint (Figure 7.17). Johnson's zone of vulnerability (Figure 7.18) demonstrates where and which bones are most likely to be damaged during the FOOSH scenario.

Scaphoid fractures (Figure 7.19, p. 124)

Initial detection of the scaphoid fracture can be difficult with failure having important ramifications for the patient. Loss of the lateral scaphoid fat strip (or its shift laterally) is a useful indicator employed when routine projections have failed to display the non-displaced scaphoid fracture. Re-examination after 10–14 days will reveal a line of new callus or bone resorption that confirms a fracture is present. Macro-radiography, radio-nuclide imaging or magnetic resonance scanning are widely suggested as alternative diagnostic tools[10–12].

Multiple complications following the scaphoid fracture include:

* avascular necrosis – the pattern of division of the vascular network at the scaphoid waist may lead to loss of blood supply after fracture (Figure 7.20, p. 124);
* long-term arthritic changes:
  ○ associated joint space loss;
  ○ sclerosis;
  ○ osteophytosis and sub-chondral cysts.

During the early stages of avascular necrosis, hyperaemia of the portion of the scaphoid that retains its blood supply causes leaching of

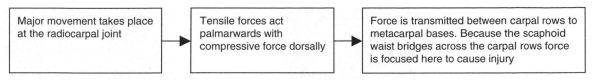

| Major movement takes place at the radiocarpal joint | → | Tensile forces act palmarwards with compressive force dorsally | → | Force is transmitted between carpal rows to metacarpal bases. Because the scaphoid waist bridges across the carpal rows force is focused here to cause injury |

Figure 7.17   Force transmission across carpal bones.

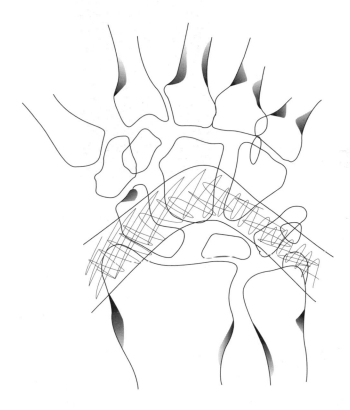

Figure 7.18   Johnson's zone of vulnerability.

bone salts to generate a porous appearance. This does not occur in the avascular portion so that the fractured segment appears whiter and more sclerotic. Later the avascular portion begins to disintegrate, allowing arthritic changes to develop. Where non-union is definite a pseudo-arthrosis is created with rounded, sclerotic bone surfaces being evident radiographically. This may be treated surgically with a bone graft and Herbert screw approach.

Other carpal bone injuries include:

- avulsion of the posterior surface of the triquetral (seen in lateral projections, Figure 7.21);
- fracture of pisiform, hook of hamate and trapezium following a direct blow;
- lunate fractures are unusual but are susceptible to avascular necrosis;
- proximal pole fractures of the hamate may follow lunate/ perilunate dislocations;

Seven

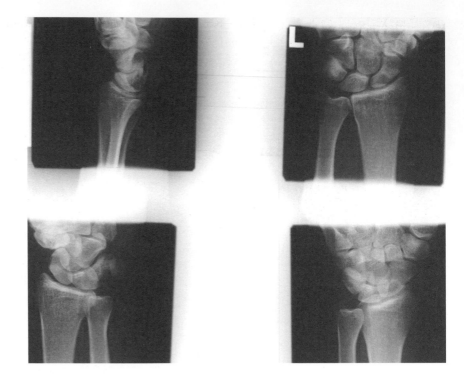

Figure 7.19 Fracture of the scaphoid waist.

Figure 7.20 Scaphoid fractures: type and the effect on blood supply (shaded area potentially compromised tissue).

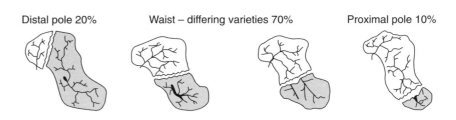

Distal pole 20%   Waist – differing varieties 70%   Proximal pole 10%

- transverse capitate fractures are usually associated with complex fracture-dislocation patterns.

Scapholunate and perilunate injuries (Figures 7.22–7.25)

The complex nature of wrist anatomy may result in a range of injuries to the ligaments as well as the bones in the following sequence.

Self-test answer

A lucency is evident across the waist of the scaphoid on more than one projection, indicating a fracture of the bone.

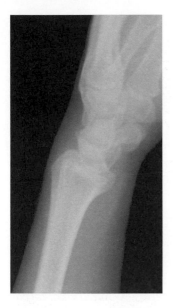

Figure 7.21 Lateral left wrist displaying triquetral avulsion.

(1) Rotary subluxation of the scaphoid (impact on the scaphoid causes the bone to rotate out of its normal relationship with the lunate) occurs following an attempt to break a backward fall.

(2) The scaphoid separates from the lunate following hyperextension with ulnar deviation. The scaphoid is foreshortened on the PA projection. The full range of injuries is best visualised on the lateral wrist radiograph.

(3) Fracture of the scaphoid may also occur.

(4) The radial intercarpal space widens relative to the ulnar side, with dislocatation of the capitate from the lunate dorsally.

(5) Further force tears or avulses the triquetral ligamentous complex.

(6) This frees the other carpus to move dorsally while leaving the lunate in place.

(7) The dislocated carpus rest on the dorsal surface of the lunate.

(8) Should the forces involved in the injury be great enough, the lunate can disarticulate by rotating volarly through 90 degrees. The capitate remains aligned with the radius but sinks proximally to the wrist.

Where large forces are involved, a trans-scaphoid perilunar dislocation may occur where the scaphoid fractures through its waist. The pattern looks like the perilunate dislocation described earlier, but the proximal half of the fractured scaphoid remains attached to the lunate

Self-test answer

A small fleck of bone is seen posterior to the dorsal corner of the lunate. Closer evaluation reveals a jig-saw fit is possible with the dorsal aspect of the triquetral, suggesting an avulsion fracture of the same.

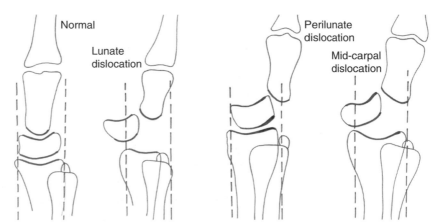

Figure 7.22 Perilunate injuries.

Seven

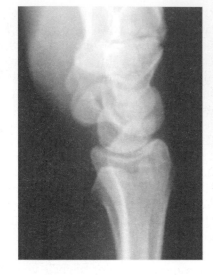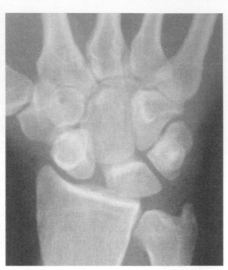

Figure 7.23   PA and lateral wrist projections showing malpositioning of the scapholunate joint.

in normal relation to the radius. Box 7.2 gives a summary of carpal dislocations.

Carpal injuries in children

When reviewing the carpal bones in the child it is wise to be aware of the order of ossification in the wrist and stages of maturity as shown in Table 7.1. It is rare to see injuries to the carpal bones before puberty although:

- the scaphoid may be injured between 10 and 15 years;
- injury tends to be at the distal pole or tubercle;
- more frequent is the dorsal avulsion fracture of the scaphoid;
- avascular problems are less frequent than in adults due to the position of scaphoid injuries; however, a creeping sclerosis or porosity may be evidence of avascular necrosis; other imaging will confirm;
- older children may display the dorsal avulsion fractures seen in adult triquetral injuries;
- the rare fracture of the lunate is detectable as a transverse line on plain films as with adult injury.

Self-test answer

The PA carpal projection shows widening of the scapholunate joint with associated shape change of the lunate. Coupled with the abnormal relationship of the radius, scaphoid, lunate and capitate on the lateral projection, this suggests a scapholunate dissociation.

Seven

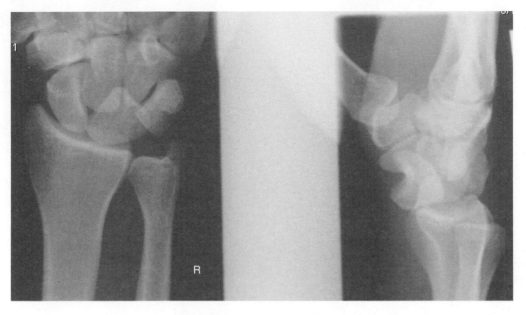

Figure 7.24   Lunate dislocation – note how the lunate has moved completely out of position on both projections.

Box 7.2   Carpal dislocations.

- Most fracture dislocations of the carpus fall within the vulnerable zone outlined by Johnson. (see Figure 7.18 p. 123).
- As scrutiny progresses from the radial to the ulnar side of the arch the injuries detected increase in **severity** but the **frequency** of injuries decreases.
- Fracture-dislocations are more common than pure dislocations.

Perilunate dislocation: The capitate articular surface is dislocated from the lunate (normally dorsally). The lunate maintains its normal articulation with the radius.

Midcarpal dislocation: The lunate tilts volarly but is not dislocated from the radius. The capitate is dislocated from the lunate but not as dorsally as in a routine perilunate dislocation.

Lunate dislocation: Lunate loses its articulation with both the capitate and radius and is displaced volarly with 90 degrees rotation. The capitate remains aligned with the radius but sinks proximally.

Self-test answer

A gross change in shape of the right lunate and overlap of the scapholunate joint suggest severe malpositioning following trauma. This is supported by the forward rotation of the lunate with associated sinking of the distal row of the carpus towards the radius. The appearance represents a lunate dislocation.

(a)

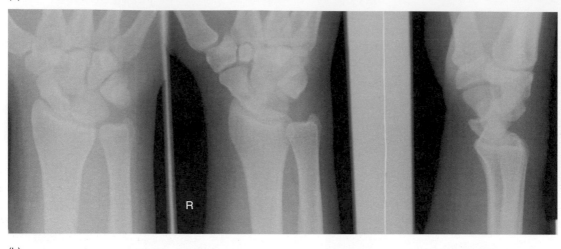

(b)

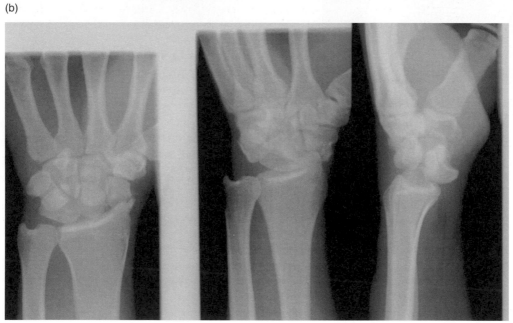

Figure 7.25 (a, b) Examples of degrees of lunate dislocation from (a) mid-carpal to (b) lunate dislocation.

Table 7.1 Order of carpal ossification in the child's wrist.*

Carpal bone	Year of appearance in wrist
Capitate	1
Hamate	2
Triquetral	3
Lunate	4
Scaphoid	5
Trapezium	6
Trapezoid	7
Pisiform†	8

*Knowledge of carpal ossification order and dates of appearance helps in the decision that a certain bone is involved in an injury according to age and gives a clue as to expected stage of skeletal maturity.
†See Figure 7.26.

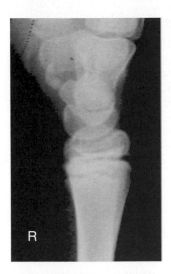

Figure 7.26 Not all is what it first appears to be – remember ossification patterns and dates. Here a pisiform is displayed in an unusual state of ossification.

Carpal dislocations are very rare in children. The lateral projection best reveals perilunar injuries with scapholunate dissociations requiring stress views in the older child, as this injury represents significant ligament damage.

Carpal instability

The normal lateral wrist radiograph displays the axes of the radius, lunate, capitate and third metacarpal base in alignment when positioned neutrally. Ligamentous injuries, because of the associated pain and loss of grip, can be detected from the relative position of these axes depending on whether the wrist is flexed or extended. Movement occurs in two main areas at the wrist, namely the lunate and radius plus the lunate and capitate in roughly equal proportions. Box 7.3 describes the final appearances on the lateral wrist projection.

With dorsal intercalated segment instability (DISI), rotary subluxation of the scaphoid can also be displayed as revealed by a scapholunate angle of 90 degrees (normal 30–60 degrees). Multiple stress-inducing projections have been devised to identify the type and extent of injury, which include flexion-extension lateral and postero-anterior (PA) projections with the fist either clenched or relaxed. More in-depth analysis of the problem is beyond the scope of this book.

Box 7.3 Pathomechanics of DISI and VISI.

Dorsiflexion
- Axis of lunate is angled dorsally relative to the axis of the radius
- Axis of capitate shows volar angulation relative to the axis of the lunate

Volar flexion
- Axis of lunate is angled volarly relative to axis of the radius
- Axis of capitate shows dorsal angulation relative to axis of lunate

DISI
or
Dorsal **I**ntercalated **S**egment **I**nstability

VISI
or
Volar **I**ntercalated **S**egment **I**nstability

Self-test answer

An unusually placed object of density similar to bone is seen anterior to the distal portion of the right scaphoid. Initially this may suggest a fracture; however, the well-corticated and rounded appearance of the bone raises the more likely suspicion that this is a variation of the normal ossification of the pisiform.

The distal radius and ulna

As already stated, the fall on the outstretched hand (FOOSH) can generate injuries that vary among the different age groups[13,14]. Typically, these can be grouped as follows:

- 4–10 years – transverse metaphyseal fracture of BOTH radius and ulna.
- 11–16 years – separation of the distal radial epiphysis.
- 17–40 years – scaphoid fractures.
- 40+ years – Colles'-type fracture.

Some features of the bony associations are worth remembering[15] (Figure 7.27a–c), as loss of the following angles can indicate an impacted fracture.

- On the PA projection, the distal radial articular surface is normally angled 17 degrees towards the ulna (Figure 7.27b).
- On the lateral projection, the distal radial articular surface is angled 10–15 degrees towards the palmar (Figure 7.27c).
- The epiphyseal scar (line) may be confused with a potential fracture appearance.
- The ulnar head at the distal radio-ulnar joint is up to 2 mm short of the radial articular surface and there may be touching or over-

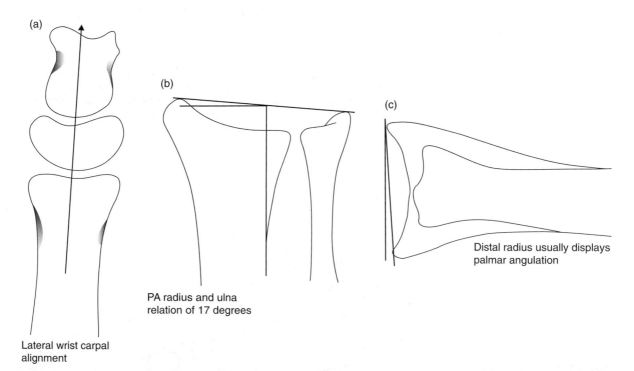

(a)

(b)

(c)

Distal radius usually displays palmar angulation

PA radius and ulna relation of 17 degrees

Lateral wrist carpal alignment

Figure 7.27a–c Normal alignment of distal radius and ulna.

lapping of the two bones (Figure 7.27c). If the ulna is shorter than the radius, this is known as negative ulnar variance. If the ulnar head lies more distally than the radius, this is positive ulnar variance. This is important for identification of distal radio-ulnar joint dislocation.

A person falling on the outstretched hand usually stresses the wrist as shown in Figure 7.28. This injury process generates the pattern typically found in the Colles-type injury of the wrist as seen in Figures 7.29 and 7.30. Most cases display:

- a transverse fracture line;
- an associated ulnar styloid avulsion injury; and
- the normal palmar angulation seen laterally is lost, often displaying a dorsal angulation of the distal fracture fragment of the radius.

Further image assessment following initiation of fracture treatment includes the following.

- Assessment of the degree of reduction related to normal angulation.
- Is the above maintained?
- Is the radiocarpal relationship intact?
- Is the distal radio-ulnar joint congruous? Its loss can cause functional disability.
- Acute carpal tunnel syndrome follows median nerve involvement.
- Disuse atrophy or reflex dystrophy (osteoporotic appearances) may be encountered with associated pain and lack of wrist use.

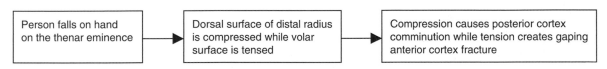

Figure 7.28 Pathomechanics of Colles' fracture.

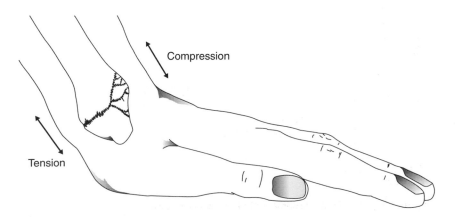

Figure 7.29 Colles' fracture generation.

Seven

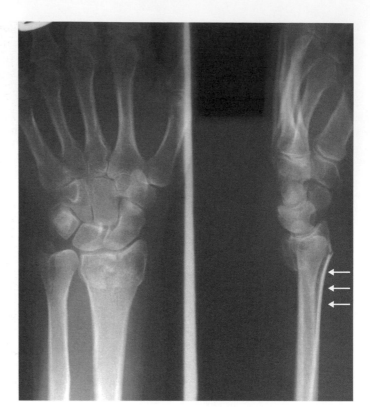

Figure 7.30 Colles'-type fracture of the right distal radius, with ulnar styloid avulsion. Arrows: location of pronator quadratus fat plane.

Usually distal radial fractures are noted within 2 cm proximal to the joint and are revealed by a soft tissue shadow in the pronator quadratus fat plane (see Figure 7.30), which may be the only evidence of an SH1 or other undisplaced fracture. An oblique projection helps confirmation of fracture.

Ulnar styloid injuries can occur in isolation and are usually the result of avulsion by the ulnar collateral and triangular fibrocartilaginous complex. They are also associated with other injury processes such as:

- epiphyseal separations;
- distal radial fractures (Figure 7.31);
- perilunate injuries of the carpal bones.

Self-test answer

A dense line is seen across the right distal radius on the PA projection with obvious impaction of fragments and loss of normal bone angulation on the lateral view. These appearances are consistent with the Colles'-type injury of the distal radius.

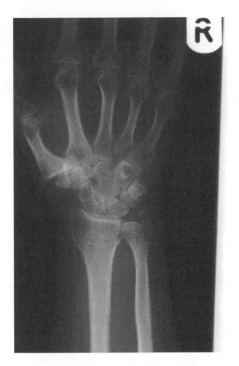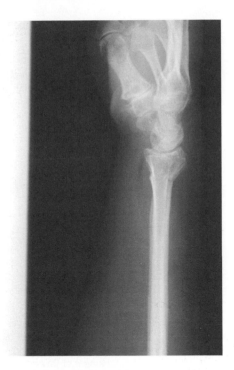

Figure 7.31   A more complex fracture of the right wrist with associated ulnar styloid avulsion.

Where the fractured ulnar styloid fails to unite following treatment, rounded, corticated bone forms that resembles a secondary ossification centre. Many eponymous descriptions have been given to fractures of the distal radius and ulna. The relationship between the eponym and the injury generated should be fully appreciated or inappropriate management may result. Eponyms that are often encountered are given in Table 7.2 and Figure 7.32.

Distal radius and ulna injuries in the child

The above injuries occur in the skeletally mature. In the under-12 age group, 35% of fractures involve the distal radius. Consistency of injury

Self-test answer

A degree of osteopenia is present. A fracture line is seen to extend across the distal radius with loss of the normal palmar angulation on the lateral projection. The ulnar styloid process is avulsed, which is indicative of a more complex injury process.

Seven

Table 7.2   Eponymous injuries of the distal radius and ulna.

Eponym	Description	Associations
Colles' fracture	Dorsal angulation of the distal radius produces the classic 'dinner-fork' deformity on the lateral radiograph Normally accompanied by an avulsed/fractured ulna styloid process	Occurs in older people Incidence rises in women between 45 and 60 years to result in six-fold more fractures in women than men Degree of post-menopausal osteoporosis dictates potential morbidity Associated hip and shoulder injuries occur in the elderly
Smith's fracture	Palmar angulation of distal radius	Occurs following impaction of a supinated forearm against a dorsi-flexed wrist Less common than Colles' but shows anterior displacement of distal fragments with palmar angulation of articular surfaces of radius
Barton's fracture	Fracture of the posterior joint margin of distal radius with proximal displacement of fragments and carpus	Usually seen in high-energy trauma such as motorcycle injuries May be noted in FOOSH injuries in the elderly Fragment size dictates stability of reduction and hence morbidity/prognosis = interior fixation
Reverse Barton's fracture	Fracture of the anterior joint margin of distal radius with proximal displacement of fragments and carpus	More common than Barton's May involve 50% or more of anterior joint surface Fragment size dictates stability of reduction and hence morbidity/prognosis = interior fixation
Hutchinson's fracture	Usually an undisplaced fracture of the radial styloid This may be an avulsion of the distal tip or an oblique or transverse fracture extending from the scapholunate joint Often a result of a direct blow	Usually seen easily on the PA projection Remember not to confuse with radial epiphyseal scar

site is remarkable, with 6–10 year olds displaying injuries in the distal radius usually in the 2–4 cm section proximal to the epiphyseal line. Other features that should be noted in the younger patient are as follows.

- Torus fractures (Greek = protuberance) display cortical bone buckling (alternative name is the buckle fracture) on the compressed side during a FOOSH injury (Figure 7.33).
- Greater forces generate a greenstick fracture where one cortex actually suffers a true fracture often with resultant fragment angulation.
- Salter–Harris fracture-dislocations of the distal epiphysis are seen in 10–16-year-old patients.
- Salter–Harris type II injuries account for around 50% of all epiphyseal injuries and are most common after the age of 10 years. Infants tend to have metaphyseal injuries.
- Often a small corner of metaphyseal bone is also included in the Salter–Harris II injuries – the corner sign. This useful indicator is

Seven

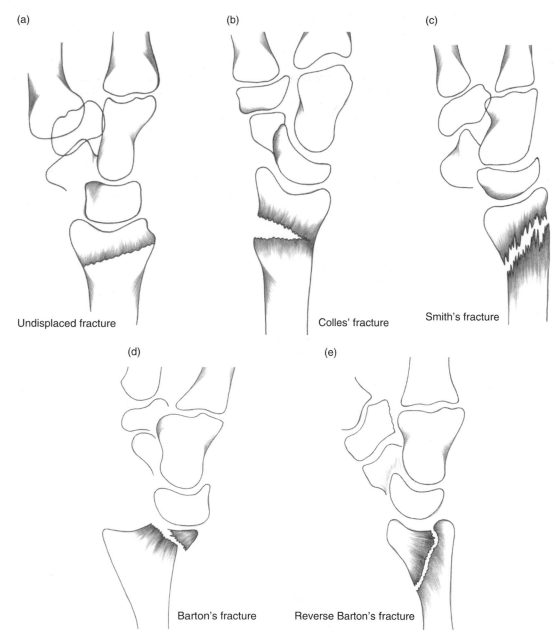

(a) Undisplaced fracture

(b) Colles' fracture

(c) Smith's fracture

(d) Barton's fracture

(e) Reverse Barton's fracture

Figure 7.32 Eponymous wrist injuries from the lateral perspective.

of prognostic value, and should be sought on the lateral wrist film (Figure 7.34)

- Torus, greenstick or separation of fracture parts may be noted in wrist injuries. When deformity is minimal, these injuries remodel well in the under-10s.

Seven

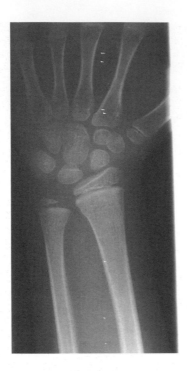 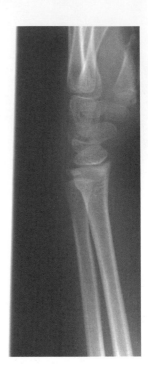

Figure 7.33 Torus fracture – left wrist.

Radius and ulna fractures

Fractures of the forearm are quite common and result from the FOOSH mechanism, compression along the long axis of the bone or from a direct blow. Forearm fracture patterns include:

- fracture of one bone;
- fracture of both bones;
- fracture of one bone with dislocation of the second.

Of these, the majority (60%) involve the middle third (Figure 7.35) with the distal and proximal thirds sharing the remaining 40% of injuries. Following these injuries those patients who present with dorsally angled fractures have a distal fracture fragment that is held in supination. Fractures that have a volar angulation result in the limb being held in

Self-test answer

A bulge on the medial border of the left radius is seen with apparent bowing of the bone towards the ulna and concomitant bulging of the lateral ulnar metaphysis towards the radius. There is also a loss of the normal bony arrangement on the lateral projection. Both projections support the diagnosis of a torus-type fracture of the distal radius with a possible bowing fracture of the ulna.

Seven

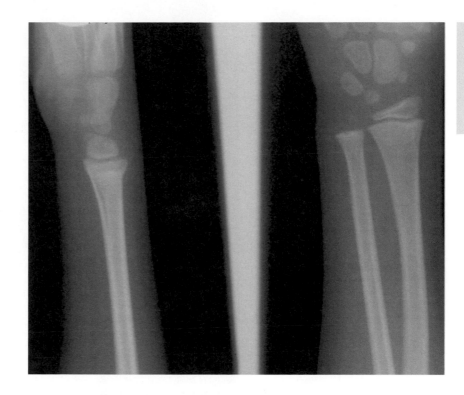

Figure 7.34 Remember to check the metaphyseal angles for the less obvious fracture.

pronation. Fractures of both bones of the forearm are frequently seen in children.

Monteggia fracture-dislocation

The ulnar shaft is fractured and there is an associated dislocation of the proximal radius. Occasionally the radial dislocation may be overlooked. In children, the ulnar component of the Monteggia lesion could be a greenstick type fracture. In these cases, radial dislocation may be noted but the fractured ulna could be missed as it presents from overt fracture to subtle bowing. Figure 7.36 shows a Monteggia fracture-dislocation compared with an anterior fracture-dislocation. See also Figure 7.37.

Self-test answer

Although no apparent change can be seen on the PA projection, a subtle sharpening of the metaphyseal angle is noted on the dorsal border of the distal radius on the lateral projection. These appearances are consistent with a metaphyseal fracture of the distal radius.

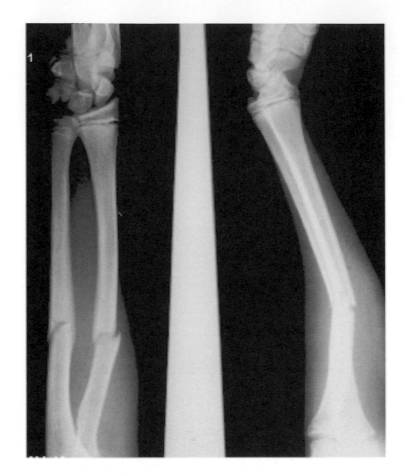

Figure 7.35 Disruption of the ring structure of the radius and ulna following mid-shaft fracture.

Galeazzi fracture-dislocation

There is usually a displaced angulated oblique middle-to-distal third fracture of the radius. As the distal radius is displaced there is disruption of the triangular fibrocartilaginous complex and subluxation of the distal radio-ulnar joint. Exercise care with the appearances here, as features of the distal lesion may not be obvious.

Nightstick fracture

This is a single injury to the mid-shaft of the ulna and is the result of a person defending themselves against a blow from above, e.g. by a base-

Self-test answer

Fractures at the proximal to middle junctions of the shafts of the radius and ulna are seen with associated dorsal angulation of the distal portions of the fragments.

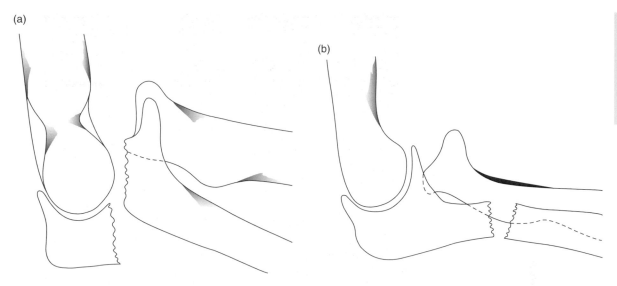

Figure 7.36 Comparison between (a) anterior fracture-dislocation and (b) the Monteggia lesion. Note the intact proximal radio-ulnar joint in (a).

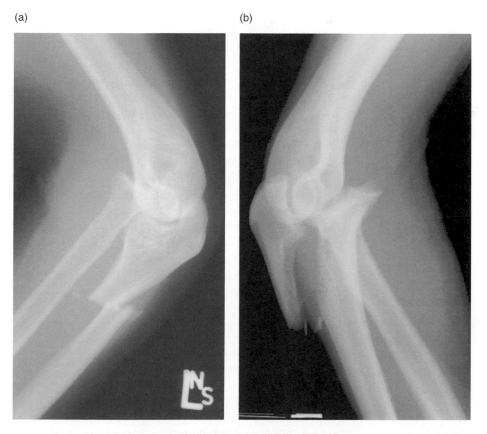

Figure 7.37 (a) Monteggia fracture pattern. Note the typical radial head dislocation with associated ulnar shaft fracture. (b) An ulnar fracture that may be misconstrued as a variation of the Monteggia pattern. (The radiocapitellar joint is still intact).

Seven

ball bat or stick. Originally called the nightstick fracture as a result of the over-zealous apprehension of a criminal by a police officer, injuries are usually found in the distal third of the ulna. The fractures tend to be transverse or slightly oblique. Associated proximal radial head dislocations should be excluded, which confirms the injury is not a Monteggia-type fracture-dislocation.

The elbow

Elbow injuries

Elbow fractures occur by the FOOSH mechanism, following a direct blow or by the pull of ligaments. The particular injury patterns are closely associated with the flexion at the elbow at the time of the insult[16]. In general, however, the following principles are usually helpful in assessing elbow trauma.

- Anterior humeral line position.
- Radiocapitellar line position.
- Fat pad elevation.
- Careful scrutiny of ossification centres is advised in the child, especially the medial epicondyle.

Normal projection shows the articulation of the radius with the capitellum of the humerus and of the ulna with the trochlea. Bowman's angle describes the carrying angle of the elbow and the normal value is 165 degrees to displace the hand away from the thigh. This angle is greater in females. The lateral projection should show the humeral condyles as being anterior to the humeral shaft. The anterior humeral line is drawn along the appropriate humeral cortex and in the normal elbow should intersect the middle third of the capitellum as seen laterally (Figure 7.38), and is useful in assessment of occult supracondylar fracture.

A second useful line that can be applied to both elbow projections is the radiocapitellar line (Figure 7.39). The cortices of the radial shaft are bisected so the line crosses the radial head to intersect the capitellum. If this does not occur in either projection, then a radial head dislocation can be inferred, and further scrutiny for associated fractures should be undertaken.

Elevation of the fat pads (Figure 7.40) becomes apparent as a result of effusion within the injured elbow. The anterior fat pad is normally seen as a straight line in the coronoid fossa but bulges anteriorly following injury, severe OA, or overflexion. In the absence of effusion the posterior fat pad cannot be seen in the olecranon fossa but becomes convex with effusions. The elevation of the posterior fat pad is a strong indicator of fracture. Fat pad elevation in children may not always be significant[17]. Radial neck fractures lie outside the joint capsule so are not usually associated with effusions or other soft tissue signs.

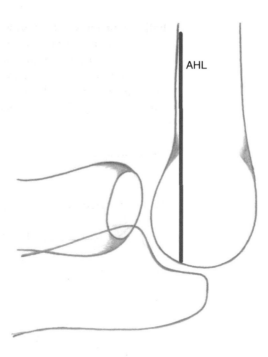

Figure 7.38 The normal anterior humeral line (AHL).

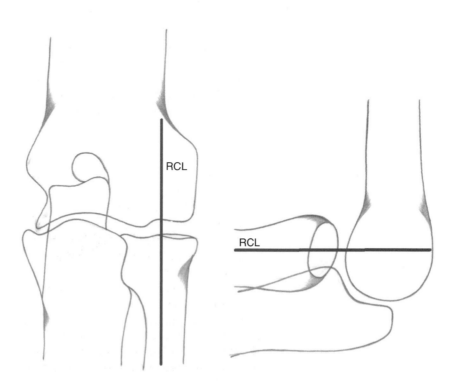

Figure 7.39 The radiocapitellar line (RCL).

Seven

(a)

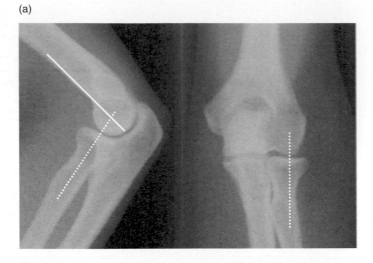

(b)

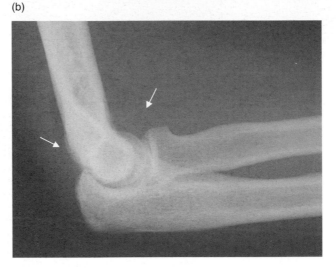

Figure 7.40 (a) The normal elbow with radiocapitellar (· · ·) and anterior humeral lines (—) superimposed. (b) The elevated fat pad sign (arrows) with associated occult fracture.

Elbow fractures in adults (Figures 7.41 and 7.42)

Most adult elbow fractures are noted in the radial head (see Figure 7.41) with an associated fat pad sign. Approximately half of these injuries are undisplaced. Where the distal humerus is fractured, detection is rarely a problem. The distribution of such injuries is as follows.

- 50% – T- or Y-shaped bicondylar fractures.
- 30% – highly comminuted T- or Y-shaped bicondylar fractures.
- 10% – capitellar fractures.
- 5% – fractures of the medial or lateral epicondyle.

The distal humeral injuries listed above have some particular features depending on the aetiology. These are summarised in Table 7.3.

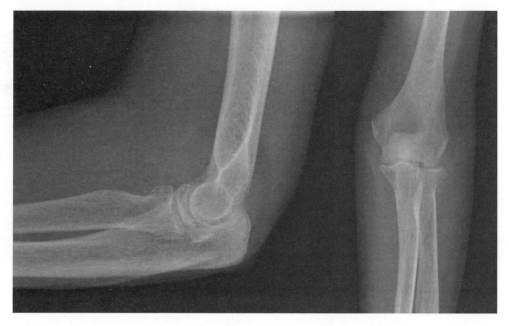

Figure 7.41   Radial head fracture.

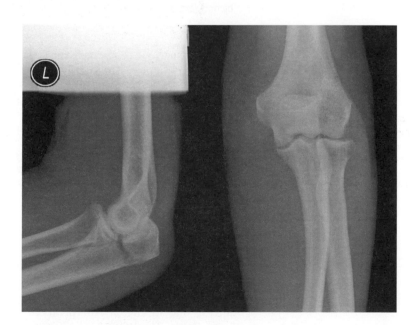

Figure 7.42   Fracture of the
olecranon following a slip on
ice to land on the flexed elbow.

Self-test answer (Figure 7.41)

A lucency on the antero-medial aspect of the radial head is seen
with associated depression of a bone fragment. Elevated fat pads
are evident consistent with a radial head fracture.

Seven

(a)   (b)

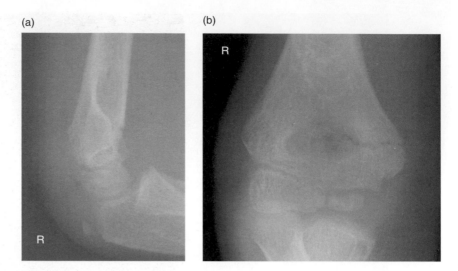

Figure 7.43 (a, b) The supracondylar fracture.

Table 7.3 Injury type and aetiology of adult elbow fractures.

Injury type	Aetiology
T- or Y-shaped bicondylar fractures	Fall on the flexed elbow in older individuals with osteoporosis Condylar fragments may be displaced and rotated by muscle pull Crushing or 'sideswipe' may cause marked comminution
Capitellar fractures	Shearing forces from radial head or lateral margin of trochlear groove may generate intra-articular capitellar fractures May be seen with radial head fracture
Medial or lateral condyle fractures	Caused by chiseling-off following direct fall onto the flexed elbow Angular force is transmitted through the trochlear notch by the ulna **or** through the capitellum by the radial head The oblique fracture generated involves one of the condyles. Stability depends upon the position of fracture line

Elbow fractures in children

Childhood elbow fractures are mainly of the supracondylar variety (Figure 7.43), accounting for approximately 60% of injuries[18], with radial head injuries predominating in the over 10's. Most show posterior displacement of the condyles/capitellum relative to the anterior humeral line in the lateral projection and display elevated fat pads (Figure 7.44). The FOOSH mechanism creates an extension force across

Self-test answer

Loss of the normal anterior humeral line relations coupled with the lucent line seen across the distal humerus led to the diagnosis of a supracondylar-type fracture of the right elbow.

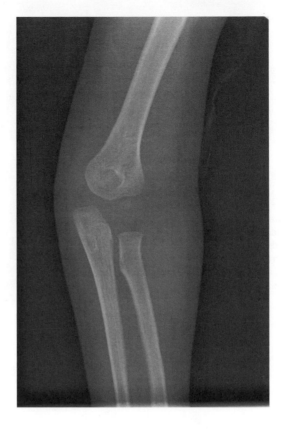

Figure 7.44 Dislocation of the left ulna – the radiocapitellar line indicates correct relationship of the lateral portion of the joint while revealing a dislocation of the juvenile ulna.

the elbow to produce a transverse fracture line through the condyles, coronoid and olecranon fossae. Occult fractures may only be revealed by an abnormal cubitus valgus or varus angulation – check Bowman's angle. Compression, distraction and cubitus varus strain on the elbow produce a radial head fracture.

Unilateral condylar fractures are seen in children:

- 15% of injuries involving the lateral epicondyle present as a Salter–Harris II injury. The extensor muscle mass causes posterior movement of the metaphyseal fragment;
- the medial epicondyle may be avulsed following exertion stresses. Failure to identify this malpositioning may result in severe disability.

Ulnar dislocations can also be seen in children (Figure 7.44).

The complexities of the development of the elbow's secondary ossification centres have led to the development of the mnemonic CRITOL (Table 7.4, Figure 7.46), which describes the order of ossification that should be expected to be present in children of different age groups. The use of this mnemonic will allow many difficult injuries to be ruled out as ossification centres may be misinterpreted incorrectly by the untrained observer. Medial epicondylar injuries (Figure 7.47) are more common as the lateral epicondyle ossifies later and fuses earlier, and the medial epicondyle is more prominent.

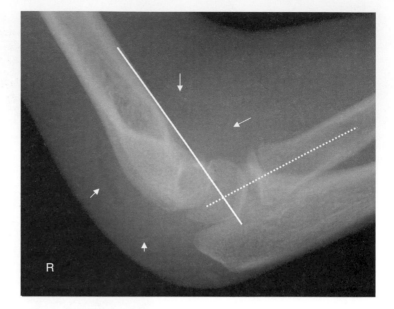

Figure 7.45 Juvenile elbow abnormality indicators in action revealing a supracondylar fracture. Superimposed lines and arrowheads are used to identify relations as in Figure 7.40.

Table 7.4 The CRITOL mnemonic.

Name of joint part	Date of appearance of ossification	Date of fusion
Capitellum	Year 1 post-natal	Fuses with **T** and **L** at puberty and joins to shaft by 15 or 16 years
Radial head	Year 4 post-natal	Fuses with radial shaft by 15 or 16 years
Internal (medial) epicondyle	Years 4–6 post-natal	Remains separate but should fuse with main bone by 20 years
Trochlea	Years 9 or 10 post-natal	Fuses with **C** and **L** at puberty and shaft by 15 or 16 years
Olecranon	Year 10 post-natal	Joins to shaft by 15 or 16 years
Lateral epicondyle	Appears by year 12	Fuses with **C** and **T** at puberty and shaft by 15 or 16 years

Self-test answer

The lateral projection of the right elbow displays strong evidence of intracapsular haematomas as evidenced by raised fat pads. The anterior humeral line indicates, by its position, that an injury is present. Combination of the two signs suggests that a supracondylar fracture of the humerus has occured.

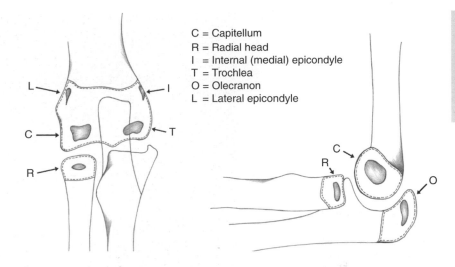

C = Capitellum
R = Radial head
I = Internal (medial) epicondyle
T = Trochlea
O = Olecranon
L = Lateral epicondyle

Figure 7.46 CRITOL.

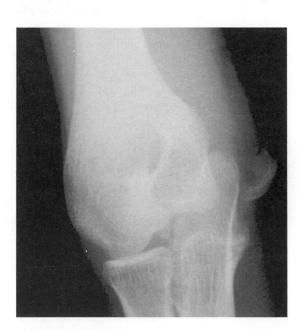

Fig 7.47 Avulsion of the right medial epicondyle.

Self-test answer

A portion of bone appears to sit in the region of the medial epicondyle of the distal right humerus. The humerus also appears to be tilted towards the radius. The appearances match those of an avulsed secondary ossification centre of the medial epicondyle.

Seven

(a)   (b)

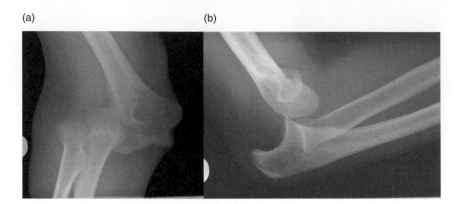

Figure 7.48   (a, b) Postero-lateral dislocation of the elbow.

Best seen on the lateral projection, radial head injuries are often of the Salter–Harris II type and many radial neck fractures are of the greenstick variety[19]. These injuries are frequently seen with other lesions caused by the FOOSH mechanism. A vertical fracture line through the radial head should also prompt a search for an associated capitellar fracture.

Proximal ulnar injuries may be caused by three distinct methods, namely the FOOSH, direct blows and avulsions. Take care not to identify the secondary ossification centre of the olecranon as an avulsion fragment. The FOOSH mechanism and direct blows cause comminution and intra-articular fracture communication.

Elbow dislocations

Most elbow dislocations show posterior or postero-lateral displacement (Figure 7.48) of the forearm bones relative to the humerus. Elbow dislocations have a strong association with local fractures. As the elbow moves out of position there may be impaction of the coronoid process or radial head resulting in a fracture. The fragments may become trapped in the joint itself. Detection of these injuries is important for the future prognostic viability of the elbow joint following reduction.

Childhood dislocations of the elbow following a FOOSH create similar injury patterns as in the adult. A posterior dislocation may induce a fracture because impaction of the coronoid process follows its collision with the trochlea. A child presenting with this problem will hold the arm flexed at 45 degrees and refuse to extend it. Occasionally,

Self-test answer

On tracing the alignment of the bone relations of the elbow it is apparent there has been a postero-lateral dislocation of the radius and ulna relative to the distal humerus.

(a)

(b)

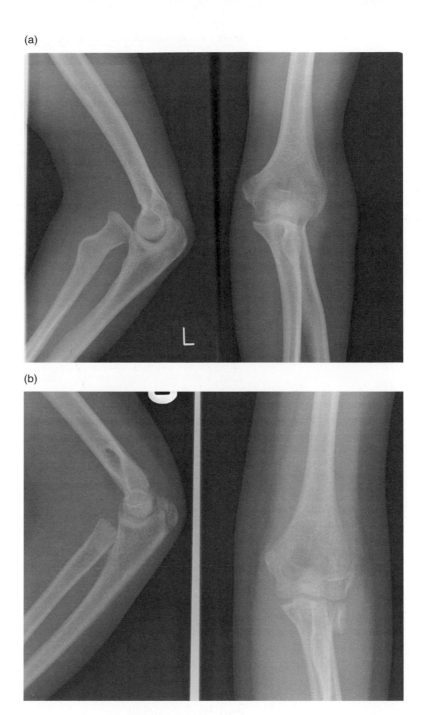

Figure 7.49 (a, b) Proximal radio-ulnar joint dislocation. In the immature skeleton the physis of the radial neck may result in weakness thus generating the pattern seen in (b). The radiograph should be scrutinised for an ulnar shaft fracture, which would indicate Monteggia injury pattern.

dislocations in other directions are seen following a direct blow to the olecranon of the flexed elbow. The radius and ulna may dislocate in opposite directions, the ulna moving posteriorly and radius anteriorly (Figure 7.49). Medial and lateral radius and ulnar dislocations are best revealed by a coronal shift as revealed on the anterior projection.

Seven

Table 7.5   Age-related shoulder girdle injuries.

Age	Injury types
Childhood	Clavicle fracture during birth
	Clavicle or proximal humeral fracture due to sport and play
20–40 years	Clavicle fracture, acromioclavicular separation and shoulder dislocation due to sport or high-energy trauma
Elderly	Neck of humerus fracture with strong pathological link to either endocrine or neoplastic metastatic disease
All ages	Humeral shaft fracture due to high-energy trauma

The shoulder girdle and proximal humerus

Shoulder injuries are common throughout life, displaying different patterns according to age and activity[20] (Table 7.5).

Clavicular fracture

This is the most common shoulder injury in childhood, 50% occurring in the under-10s and 90% as a result of the FOOSH mechanism generating force through the shoulders. Most clavicular fractures heal without incident; however, acro-osteolysis (resorption of the end of the clavicle distal to the fracture following trauma) may be seen as a result of these injuries.

- Undisplaced fractures of medial third (and occasionally mid-third) may be difficult to visualise without cephalic angulation as the fracture often overlies the ribs.
- Middle third is involved in 65–80% of fractures, which are normally transverse and sometimes comminuted (Figure 7.50).
- Infrequently, severe trauma causes mid-clavicular fracture with vascular injury or less commonly injury to the brachial plexus. Least commonly, the axillary artery is injured.
- The outer third is involved in 15–30% of fractures and it is suggested these should be stressed to confirm the integrity of the coracoclavicular ligaments (Figure 7.51).

Acromioclavicular joint injuries (Figure 7.52)

These account for 12% of all shoulder dislocations.

- These are common sports injuries, caused by a direct fall on the shoulder or indirectly by a FOOSH.
- Usually occur between the ages of 15 and 40 years and are rare in childhood.

Seven

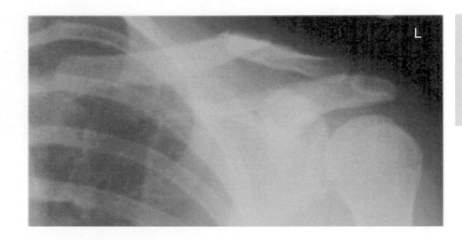

Figure 7.50 Mid-clavicular fracture of left shoulder.

- Normal acromioclavicular joint space varies from 3 to 5 mm with occasional ones as large as 7 mm. Normal alignment should be scrutinised.
- The difference between an individual's acromioclavicular joint dimensions should not be more than 2 mm. Where this is not the case, comparison views of the two sides are advised.

A sequence of events outlining the likely appearances of acromioclavicular and coracoclavicular ligament damage in shoulder injuries is shown in Figure 7.53. The coracoclavicular and acromioclavicular ligaments are shown in Figure 7.54.

Sternoclavicular joint injuries

Sternoclavicular joint dislocations are rare entities accounting for approximately 3% of shoulder girdle dislocations.

- Anterior dislocation is the usual pattern, with road traffic accidents and sporting injuries accounting for the majority of presentations. The sternal end of the clavicle presents as a bulbous protuberance.
- Posterior dislocation of the clavicle prevents palpation of its medial end.
- Neurovascular damage may occur.
- High-energy impacts are frequent causes of injury so chest radiographs should be scrutinised for pneumothoraces. Tracheal or oesophageal rupture may be associated with sternoclavicular

Self-test answer

Loss of the normal presentation of alignment of the left mid-clavicle suggests a fracture with depression of the lateral portion.

Seven

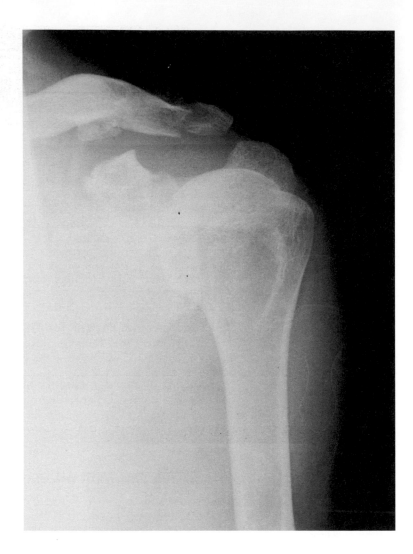

Figure 7.51 Fracture of the outer third of the clavicle may be associated with coraco- or acromioclavicular ligament rupture. In this case there is the impression of an associated coracoid process fracture.

dislocation. Tracheal pressure can cause breathing difficulties and a voice change following impingement of the laryngeal nerve.

Detection of sternoclavicular dislocation on plain films is notoriously difficult and computed tomography (CT) should be considered to confirm the diagnosis.

The scapula (Figure 7.55)

The protection offered to the scapula by a relatively thick muscle layer means the scapula is rarely injured. However, when it is damaged violent forces are involved and as such scapular fractures often accompany potentially life-threatening injuries such as:

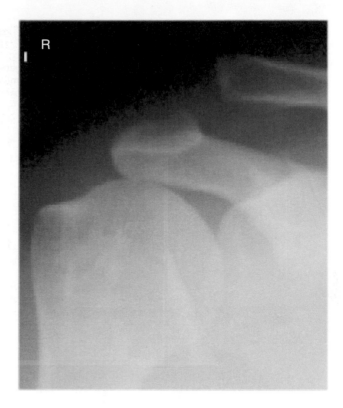

Figure 7.52 Right acromioclavicular joint disruption.

- cerebral contusions;
- skull fractures;
- rib fractures;
- clavicular fractures;
- lung or pulmonary damage;
- brachial plexus injury;
- vertebral fractures;
- pelvic fractures;
- fracture or dislocation of the extremities.

Epileptic fits or electric shocks also have an association with scapular fractures. Most scapular injuries are manifested as acromion and coracoid process fractures with glenohumeral or acromioclavicular dislocations.

Self-test answer

Complete loss of the normal association of the right acromio-clavicular joint suggests soft tissue injury. The degree of displacement of the bony components suggests involvement of both the acromio- and coracoclavicular ligamentous structures.

Injuries occur in sequence relative to force applied:

- Sprain or tear of acromioclavicular ligaments
- Sprain or tear of coracoclavicular ligaments
- Detachment of deltoid or trapezius muscles from the clavicle
- Intra-articular fracture of acromion or clavicle, fracture of coracoid process

This produces, relative to the degree of force involved:

- Widening of the acromioclavicular joint
- Superior clavicular displacement following tearing of the coracoclavicular ligaments

Any or all of the following will be seen on the film:

- Widening of the acromioclavicular joint
- Presence or absence of vertical clavicular displacement
- Vertical displacement of outer end of clavicle at acromioclavicular joint

Figure 7.53
Acromioclavicular joint injuries related to force application.

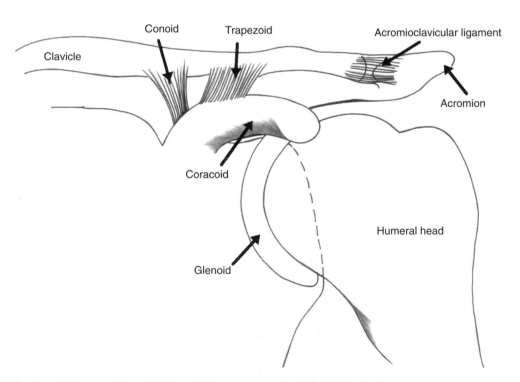

Figure 7.54 The coraco- and acromioclavicular ligaments. Note the coracoclavicular ligament is formed from the conoid and trapezoid ligaments that rupture according to the degree of force applied.

(a) (b)

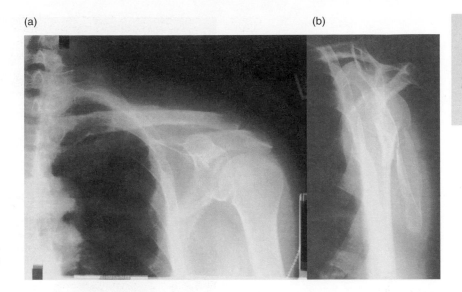

Figure 7.55 (a) AP and (b) Y-view lateral of the fractured left scapula.

Where fractures occur following major trauma, the majority of injuries (80%) are in the scapular body. Avulsion injuries are seen at the following sites:

- acromion;
- coracoid;
- glenoid (inferior margin);
- inferior angle of scapula;
- superior and lateral borders of the scapula.

Ossification of the inferior angle of the scapula can be confused with avulsive injury, and nutrient canals misinterpreted as fractures. Adolescents often show avulsion of the triceps insertion at the base of the glenoid following throwing movements. The coracoid process may be fractured at its base following acromioclavicular dislocation or, rarely, following a direct blow. Multiple ossification centres in adolescents are often confused with avulsion fractures.

Proximal humerus fractures

There are two main stages of life when proximal humeral fractures are encountered. These are:

- under 20 years;
- following the menopause where women show a threefold greater incidence compared with men.

Major trauma is the commonest cause of injury in the 20–45 year age group. Shoulder dislocation is the most frequent association in these cases. In anterior and posterior dislocations, 15% display avulsion of the greater tuberosity of humerus.

Seven

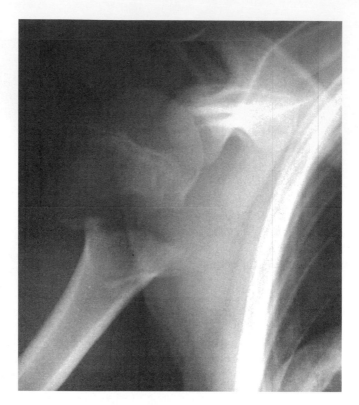

Figure 7.56 Juvenile humeral neck fracture of the right side. Pathological fractures of this area are often associated with simple cystic lesions of the humeral neck.

Most fractures of the proximal humerus involve the anatomical or surgical neck with an associated greater or lesser tuberosity fracture. The components of the fracture usually impact through the surgical neck as displacement of the fragments does not always occur. However, muscle and tendinous pull causes rotation of the humeral head and, occasionally, fragment displacement that may require open reduction and fixation (Figure 7.56).

Humeral shaft fractures may occur for several reasons, including:

* moderate trauma (from falls);
* direct blows;
* severe trauma (e.g. road traffic accident);
* throwing exertion;
* torsional strains such as when using exercise equipment, shot putting or arm wrestling.

Nerve injury is seen in approximately a fifth of cases. As the humerus is a long bone, all types of fracture are noted with the location and direction of the fracture line being dictated by the strength and directions of the applied force. Table 7.6 describes the aetiology and predominance of the different fracture types.

Table 7.6 Humeral fracture: types, aetiology and predominance.

Fracture type	Aetiology	Position of fracture	Predominance (%)
Transverse fractures*	Angled humeral shaft at time of injury	Mid-third	70
Oblique and spiral fractures	Torsional forces are transmitted through the humerus	Proximal and middle third junction	10
Comminuted fracture	Combination of above with higher energy	Distal and middle third junction	10
		Proximal third	<5
		Distal third	<7

*Transverse fractures with a pathological cause other than osteoporosis usually pass through the disease focus. Myeloma or metastatic breast deposits are usual causes in adults while bone cysts in the proximal humeral shaft may act as the focus in children.

Glenohumeral dislocation

The shoulder is the most commonly dislocated joint, accounting for approximately 50% of all dislocations. Eighty-five per cent of shoulder dislocations are glenohumeral, while childhood injury is rare. Where anterior dislocation occurs there may be recurrent dislocation in about 40% of cases; however, this falls with increasing age at initial injury. Anterior dislocations are usually seen in the following order of frequency:

- sub-coracoid;
- sub-glenoid;
- sub-clavicular;
- intrathoracic.

Usually, anterior dislocation is generated by external rotation of the abducted arm. Impaction of the postero-lateral surface of the humeral head on the glenoid rim may cause a compression fracture to generate the Hill–Sachs deformity. Damage to the glenoid labrum (and hence the capsulo-ligamentous complex) produces an unstable shoulder and the Bankhart lesion[21]. This may only be detected by use of cross-sectional imaging modalities, ultrasound or arthrography/arthroscopy unless a bony component is also apparent. Approximately 15% of anterior dislocations have an associated greater tuberosity fracture that may need internal fixation if the fragment remains displaced[22].

Figure 7.57 shows a normal AP shoulder diagram. When evaluating the radiographic examination for shoulder dislocation the following questions must be answered.

- What is the final position of the humeral head?
- Has there been a glenoid or greater tuberosity fracture?
- Does the humeral head show evidence of a compression fracture?

Seven

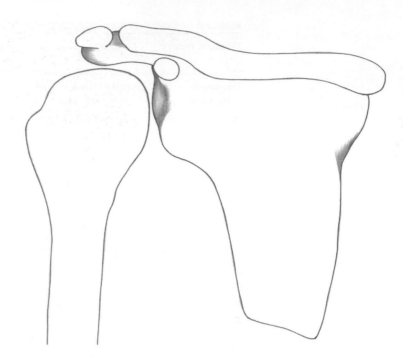

Figure 7.57   The normal AP
shoulder projection.

Compression fractures are usually evident as an indistinct line on
the lateral border of the humeral head on the externally rotated antero-
posterior projection. Internally rotated films will reveal a notch in the
lateral border. Internally and externally rotated films viewed simultane-
ously will show a vertical sclerotic line in the humeral head that marks
the medial extent of the lesion.

The axillary profile (scapulohumeral arch, Figure 7.58) on the antero-
posterior projection is a helpful way of ascertaining the direction of the
dislocation:

- bulbous distortions inferiorly indicate likely anterior dislocation;
- sharply angled axillary profile indicates likely posterior dislocation;
- chronic disease or acute rotator cuff injury (Figure 7.59) will
  display a loss of subacromion space. Sclerosis and osteophytosis
  will also be present in the chronic presentation.

Posterior dislocation usually occurs following forced posterior movement of the internally rotated humeral head[23]. Bilateral injury is seen in
convulsive disorders[24]. Falls on or direct blows to the internally rotated
and extended arm account for the remaining dislocations. Features
include:

- compression fractures of the humeral head;
- posterior glenoid rim fracture;
- lesser tuberosity avulsion injuries;

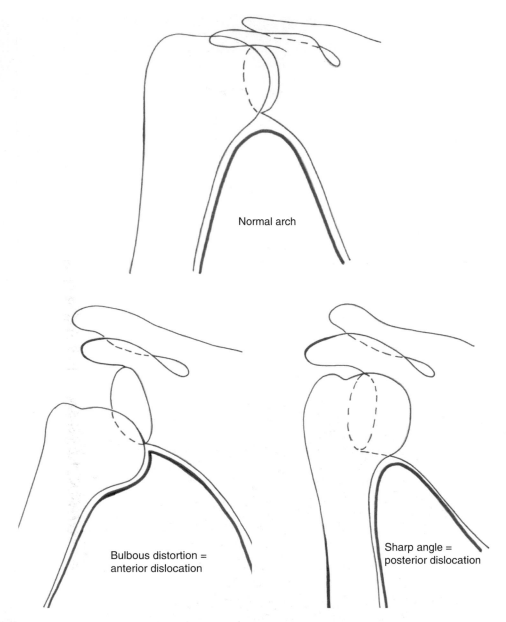

Normal arch

Bulbous distortion =
anterior dislocation

Sharp angle =
posterior dislocation

Figure 7.58   Scapulohumeral arches.

- the over-50s age group more commonly have the latter injury;
- fits/seizures are the main cause of adult posterior dislocation.

A large proportion of posteriorly dislocated shoulders (over half) are initially undetected with the loss of function being misdiagnosed. The association of posterior dislocation with lesser tuberosity fracture may detract the viewer's eye from a more significant underlying injury. This

Seven

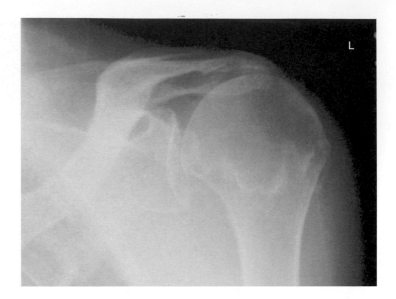

Figure 7.59 Usually a chronic disorder, rotator cuff disruption may be noted following a fall.

can also be seen in anterior dislocations (Figure 7.60). The posteriorly dislocated shoulder (Figure 7.61) is not easily differentiated on just the single antero-posterior projection. Confirmation should be sought by use of:

- the Grashey projection (anteriorly rotated AP-type projection that brings the glenoid perpendicular to the film and foreshortens the clavicle), which displays a clear glenohumeral joint space unless posterior dislocation is evident;
- an axillary view obtained infero-superiorly or in the reverse direction;
- Y-view of scapula (Figure 7.62);
- modified axial projections.

The standard AP projection can be helpful since it can show appearances suggestive of posterior dislocation.

- Humeral head is in fixed internal rotation (the light bulb appearance).
- Lateral displacement may be evident as a widened joint space (0–6 mm is the accepted normal range for glenohumeral joint space).

Self-test answer

There is an appearance of a sclerotic line around the humeral neck matching the insertion of the articular capsule. There is also an associated superior drift of the humeral head relative to the inferior surface of the acromion process of the scapula. These appearances indicate rotator cuff impingement syndrome.

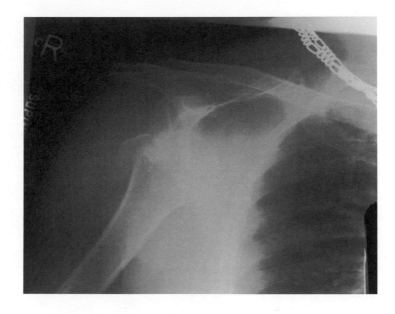

Figure 7.60 Frequently a fracture may be associated with humeral dislocation – in this case it is the lesser tuberosity.

- There is no half-moon overlap of the posterior glenoid rim and medial margin of the humeral head.

With the other projections (Figure 7.63):

- axillary views show the humeral head to be posterior with a compression notch evident on the anterior humeral head;
- Y-view shows the humeral head to be posterior relative to the glenoid, resting inferior to the acromion.

In the patient who is unable to abduct the arm, internal rotation of the humerus due to pain will create the 'light bulb' effect. This appearance strongly mimics the posterior dislocation presentation and should not be accepted as the definitive image for diagnosis without confirmation using a projection in an axial or modified axial plane.

Inferior and superior dislocation of the humeral head can also occur. In the condition luxatio erecta, the head of the humerus points inferiorly with the arm held in full abduction to allow the hand to rest on the head. In superior dislocation the humeral head is displaced through the joint capsule and rotator cuff and rests beneath the acromion. Rarely simultaneous bilateral dislocations have been reported following convulsive causes.

Self-test answer

An antero-inferior sub-coracoid dislocation of the humerus is seen. The appearances also suggest a fracture of the lesser tuberosity of the humerus that is displaced slightly inferiorly.

Seven

(a)   (b)

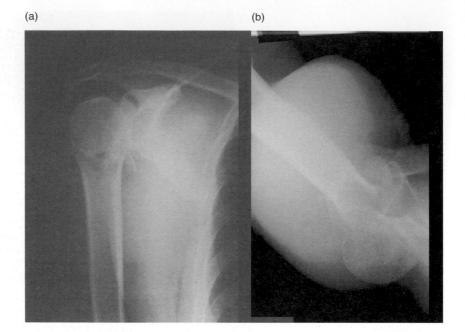

Figure 7.61   (a, b)   A posteriorly dislocated shoulder with fracture of the humeral neck. On its own the posterior dislocation is the most frequently misdiagnosed shoulder dislocation that, as a result, has the most serious consequences.

Childhood concerns

Fractures and dislocations of the clavicle feature most frequently among childhood shoulder injuries.

- Clavicular fractures tend to be seen in the under-10s with an accompanying drop of the shoulder. This may be a greenstick variety of the middle third.
- The medial end of the fracture moves cranially and the lateral portion inferiorly. About 5% of fractures of the clavicle occur in the outer third.
- Movement in clavicular fractures depends on the integrity of the coracoclavicular ligaments. Intact ligaments denote minimal displacement.

Acromioclavicular ligaments are usually ruptured by moderate local trauma while severe trauma tends to damage the coracoclavicular ligaments. Where the coracoclavicular ligaments are torn the lateral part of

Self-test answer

The appearances on the antero-posterior image are of internal rotation of the humerus with an associated fracture of the surgical neck. The axial projection reveals the humeral head to be resting posterior to the glenoid of the scapula.

(a) (b)

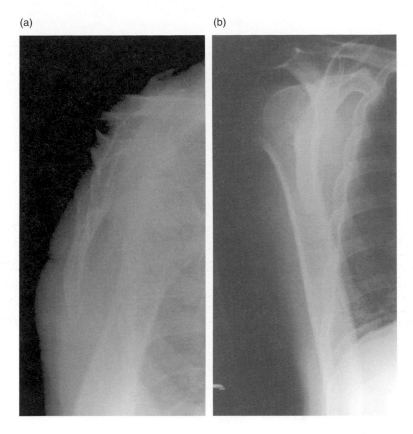

Figure 7.62 The Y projection of the scapula can be used to reveal the position of the humerus relative to the glenoid following dislocation. (a) Anterior dislocation. (b) Posterior dislocation with humeral neck fracture.

the clavicle can drift cranially. Acromioclavicular dislocations may be described as three levels, similar to the 'Tossy' classification in adults.

- Type 1 – spraining of the acromioclavicular ligaments with no movement.
- Type 2 – acute tearing of the acromioclavicular ligaments with intact coracoclavicular ligaments. May show minimal malalignment with displacement of the acromioclavicular joint up to half of the thickness of the clavicle.
- Type 3 – coracoid process avulsion fragments may accompany tearing of both sets of ligaments. The acromioclavicular joint is widened with riding of the clavicle laterally to rest above the acromion process. There will be asymmetry of the coracoclavicular space.

Significant direct force is necessary to cause injury to the scapula and even then may be of little significance unless accompanied by evidence of intrathoracic damage. Direct blows to the shoulder may generate scapular neck fractures without humeral neck injury. A vertically directed force may fracture the acromion. Secondary ossification centres of the lateral aspect of the acromion appearing during 15–18 years may be confused with fractures.

Seven

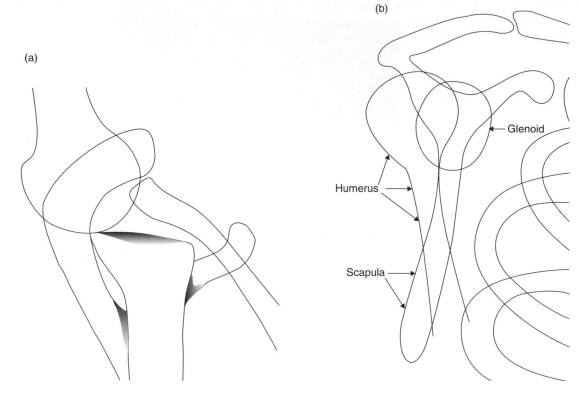

(a)

(b)

Glenoid

Humerus

Scapula

Figure 7.63 (a) Axillary and (b) Y-view projections for posterior shoulder dislocations.

Glenohumeral dislocation is rare in the immature skeleton as the growth plate forms a natural line of weakness and will transmit any force to generate a Salter–Harris type of injury.

- Birthing trauma may be considered as physeal plate slippage rather than dislocation.
- Infants tend to display Salter–Harris I injuries and Salter–Harris II injuries predominate in older children.
- If the medial growth plate of the proximal humerus is injured, early fusion may ensue with limb length problems and development of potential varus deformity.
- Occasionally, however, dislocation does occur with the majority (97%) being in an anterior direction and ending in a sub-coracoid position.
- The FOOSH is the most frequent mechanism of injury. Posterior dislocation is rarely seen leading to problems with identification.
- Shoulder point blows and non-accidental causes account for other injuries to the proximal humerus.
- Direct trauma will cause mid-shaft humeral fractures that frequently have an open wound associated with them.

- Indirect forces generate transverse, oblique and spiral fractures.
- A quarter of injuries may have associated elbow, shoulder or claviclular damage.

Seven

References

1 Angermann, P. and Lohmann, M. (1993) Injuries to the hand and wrist – a study of 50,272 injuries. *Journal of Hand Surgery (British Volume)* **18**(5), 642–4.
2 Burke, T. (1997) The radiography of shoulder dislocations. *Radiologic Technology* **69**(2), 171–2.
3 De Jonge, J.J., Kingma, J., van der Lei, B., *et al.* (1994) Phalangeal fractures of the hand. An analysis of gender and age related incidence and aetiology. *Journal of Hand Surgery (British Volume)* **19**(2), 168–70.
4 Street, J.M. (1993) Radiographs of phalangeal fractures: importance of the internally rotated oblique projection for diagnosis. *American Journal of Roentgenology* **160**(3), 575–6.
5 De Smet, L. and Stofflen, D. (1997) Clenched fist injury: a pitfall for patients and surgeons. *Acta Orthopaedica Belgica* **63**(2), 113–17.
6 Braakman, K., Verburg, A.D. and Oderwald, E.E. (1996) Are routine radiographs during conservative treatment of fractures of the fourth and fifth metacarpals useful? *Acta Orthopaedica Belgica* **62**(3), 151–5.
7 Eyres, K.S. and Allen, T.R. (1993) Skyline view of the metacarpal head in the assessment of the human fight-bite injuries. *Journal of Hand Surgery (British Volume)* **18**(1), 43–4.
8 Stapczynski, J.S. (1991) Fracture of the base of the little finger metacarpal: importance of the 'ball catcher' radiographic view. *Journal of Emergency Medicine* **9**(3), 145–9.
9 Cohen, M.S. (1997) Fractures of the carpal bones. *Hand Clinics* **13**(4), 587–99.
10 Gaebler, C., Kukla, C., Breitenseher, M.J., *et al.* (1998) Limited diagnostic value of macro radiography in suspected scaphoid fractures. *Acta Orthopedica Scandinavica* **69**(4), 401–03.
11 Kitsis, C., Taylor, M., Chandey, J., *et al.* (1998) Imaging the problem scaphoid. *Injury* **29**(7), 515–20.
12 Tiel van Buul, M.M., van Beek, E.J., Borm, J.J., *et al.* (1993) The value of radiographs and bone scintigraphy in suspected scaphoid fracture. A statistical analysis. *Journal of Hand Surgery (British Volume)* **18**(3), 403–06.
13 Hemenway, D., Azrael, D.R., Rimm, E.B., *et al.* (1994) Risk factors for wrist fracture: effect of age, cigarettes, alcohol, body height, relative weight and handedness on the risk for distal forearm fractures. *American Journal of Epidemiology* **140**(4), 361–7.
14 Hill, C., Riaz, M., Mozzam, A., *et al.* (1998) A regional audit of hand and wrist injuries. A study of 4873 injuries. *Journal of Hand Surgery (British Volume)* **23**(2), 196–200.

15 Schreibman, K.L., Freeland, A., Gilula, L.A., *et al.* (1997) Imaging of the hand and wrist. *Orthopedic Clinics of North America* 28(4), 537–82.

16 Amis, A.A. and Miller, J.H. (1995) The mechanisms of elbow fractures: an investigation using impact tests *in vitro*. *Injury* 26(3), 163–8.

17 Donnelly, L.F., Klostermeier, T.T. and Klostermeier, L.A. (1998) Traumatic elbow effusions in paediatrics: are occult fractures the rule? *American Journal of Roentgenology* 171(1), 243–5.

18 Skaggs, D. and Pershad, J. (1997) Paediatric elbow trauma. *Paediatric Emergency Care* 13(6), 425–34.

19 Sessa, S., Lascombes, P., Prevot, J., *et al.* (1996) Fractures in the radial head and associated injuries in children. *Journal of Paediatric Orthopaedics Part B* 5(3), 200–09.

20 Nordquist, A. and Petersson, C.J. (1995) Incidence and causes of shoulder girdle injuries in an urban population. *Journal of Shoulder and Elbow Surgery* 4(2), 107–12.

21 Mizuno, K., Nabeshima, Y. and Hirohata, K. (1993) Analysis of Bankhart lesion in the recurrent dislocation or subluxation of the shoulder. *Clinical Orthopaedics and Related Research* 288, 158–65.

22 Taylor, D.C. and Arciero, R.A. (1997) Pathologic changes associated with shoulder dislocations. Arthroscopic and physical examination findings in first time, traumatic anterior dislocations. *American Journal of Sports Medicine* 25(3), 306–11.

23 Berg, E.E. (1995) Posterior shoulder (gleno humeral) dislocation. *Orthopaedic Nursing* 14(1), 47–9.

24 Elberger, S.T. and Brody, G. (1995) Bilateral posterior shoulder dislocations. *American Journal of Emergency Medicine* 13(3), 331–2.

Skeletal Trauma of the Lower Limb

Renata Eyres

Introduction

Plain film radiographs are the main diagnostic tool for lower limb injuries, several of which are subtle and easily overlooked. It is therefore important to have sound knowledge and understanding of normal radiographic anatomy and the mechanism of injury in lower limb trauma.

Foot injuries

The foot can be divided into three sections:

- hindfoot – calcaneum and talus;
- midfoot – navicular, cuboid and cuneiforms;
- forefoot – metatarsals and phalanges.

Numerous accessory ossicles may be present and these can resemble fractures, such as the os trigonum (posterior to the talus), os perineum (adjacent to the cuboid) and os tibiale externum (adjacent to the navicular). Remember they are well rounded and corticated to differentiate them from fractures (see Appendix 2).

Hindfoot trauma

Talus

The most serious fractures are those that pass through the neck of the talus and although rare, these are important as they are prone to non-union and avascular necrosis[1]. **Osteochondral fractures** can be subtle and

167

Eight

may be identified by the presence of a small flake of bone fragment within the joint or a defect in the cortex of the talar dome[8]. In minor fractures of the talus a small flake of bone may become detached from the margin of an articular surface.

Calcaneum/os calcis

The majority of tarsal fractures occur in the calcaneum, the largest of the tarsal bones, of which 75% are intra-articular and 25% extra-articular[3]. The fractures may be isolated cracks with minimal displacement and usually occur in the region of the tuberosity. More common are compression injuries caused by a fall from a height – although these can also result from a simple twisting injury. These fractures are often bilateral, and associated injuries include compression fractures of the lower dorsal/upper lumbar spine.

A subtle impacted fracture of the calcaneum may be represented by a sclerotic line. The lateral view is the most helpful, although if a fractured calcaneum is clinically suspected an axial view should be obtained. A calcaneal fracture may only become apparent when assessing Bohler's angle, which is normally between 30 and 40 degrees (Figure 8.1)[4]. To calculate Bohler's angle draw a line (i) from the posterior aspect of the calcaneum to its highest mid-point and (ii) from this point to the highest point anteriorly (Figure 8.2). An angle of less than 30 degrees indicates a fracture; the smaller the angle the greater the compression, resulting in a higher risk of further complications. Late complications include osteoarthritis, stiffness in the mid- and sub-talar joint and a possible limp due to the proximal displacement of the calcaneal tuberosity. **Remember**, however, that a normal Bohler's angle does not exclude a fracture. The trabecular pattern within the calcaneum is normally well-defined. Any disruption of this pattern may indicate a subtle fracture.

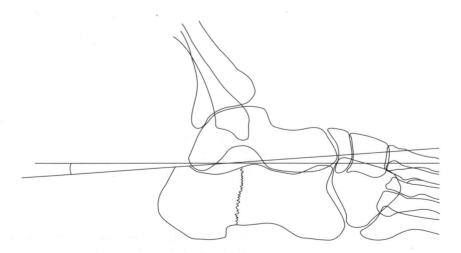

Figure 8.1 Fractured calcaneum – Bohler's angle is reduced.

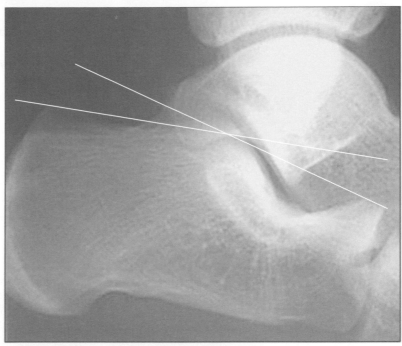

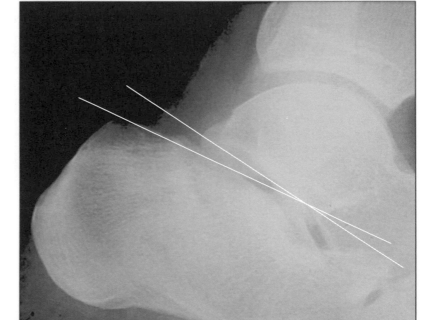

Figure 8.2 (a,b) The use of Bohler's angle to detect a calcaneal fracture.

Self-test answer

In the lateral projection figure in 8.2b detection of a calcaneal fracture is only evident from Bohler's angle which is <30 degrees.

Eight

Midfoot trauma

Tarso-metatarsal dislocation (Lisfranc injury)

This is an uncommon injury which can be easily overlooked. Thorough knowledge of the normal radiographic anatomy and alignment of the tarsal bones with the metatarsals is therefore vital.

- **Normal dorsi-palmar (DP) view** – shows that the medial margin of the second metatarsal aligns with the medial margin of the middle cuneiform.
- **Oblique projection** – shows that the medial margin of the third metatarsal aligns with the medial margin of the lateral cuneiform.

The fracture-dislocation (Figures 8.3 and 8.4) is caused by severe trauma, usually by forced inversion or eversion of the forefoot when the

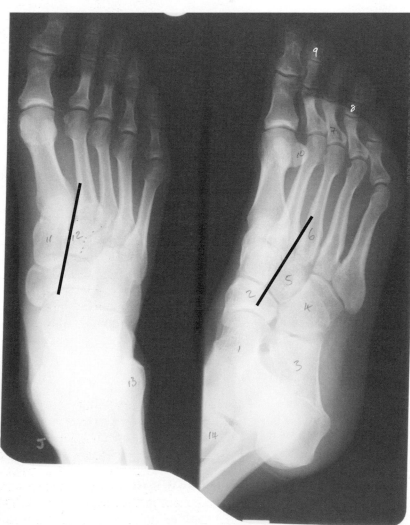

Figure 8.3   Normal anatomy and alignment of the foot. On the DP projection (left hand image) the medial aspect of the base of the second metatarsal should be aligned with the medial aspect of the medial cuneiform. On the DP oblique projection (right hand image), normal midfoot alignment is indicated when the medial aspect of the third metatarsal is aligned with the medial aspect of the lateral cuneiform. Key = talus (1); navicular (2); calcaneum (3); cuboid (4); lateral cuneiform (5); third metatarsal (6); third proximal phalanx (7); fourth middle phalanx (8); second distal phalanx (9); lateral (fibular) sesamoid bone (10); medial cuneiform (11); middle cuneiform (12); lateral malleolus (fibula) (13); tibia (14).

(a) (b)

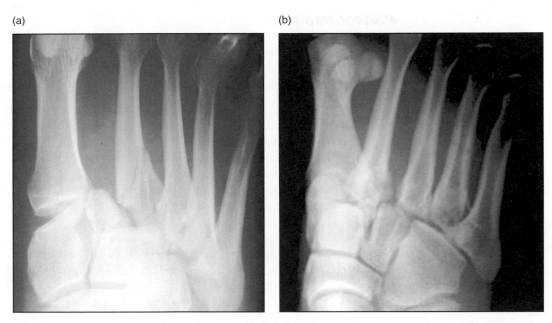

Figure 8.4 Disruption of the tarso-metatarsal joint in the Lisfranc fracture-dislocation on the (a) dorso-palmar (DP) and (b) DP oblique projections.

hindfoot is fixed. It can also occasionally be due to a crush injury. Common examples of the causes of this injury are a rider falling from a horse, with the foot stuck in the stirrup, and trapping of feet under pedals or seats in head-on road traffic accidents[5,6].

If a bony fragment is detached from the base of any of the four medial metatarsals, a tarso-metatarsal dislocation should be suspected. Occasionally a fracture of the second metatarsal occurs at a more proximal level and the base remains in normal alignment. The distal fragment then dislocates laterally with the third, fourth and fifth metatarsals. The malalignment is then usually only seen on the oblique view.

Self-test answer (Figure 8.4a)

There is an apparent disruption to the alignment of the medial margin of the second metatarsal with the medial border of the middle cuneiform. There is an oblique fracture of the base of the second metatarsal with an evident shift laterally of the metatarsals as a unit typical of the homolateral Lisfranc fracture-dislocation.

Eight

Forefoot trauma

Metatarsal injuries

These have three main causes[7].

- Direct injury caused by a heavy object falling onto the foot, e.g. fractured metatarsal shafts. One or more metatarsal shafts may be involved. The fracture may occur at any point along the shaft and is usually transverse or oblique with minimal displacement.
- Twisting injuries, e.g. fractured base of fifth metatarsal. A common twisting injury is forced inversion such as stepping awkwardly off a kerb. An avulsion fracture, where the base of the fifth metatarsal is 'pulled off' by the tendon of the peroneus brevis muscle, is the most common outcome of such an injury. However, occasionally a Jones' fracture occurs. This is a transverse fracture of the base of the fifth metatarsal (Figure 8.5), approximately 1.5–2 cm distal to the tuberosity[8].

  It is important not to confuse the transverse fracture line with an unfused apophysis, where the line is parallel to the long axis of the fifth metatarsal. An accessory ossicle, the os vesalianum, is related to the base of the fifth metatarsal but its well-corticated margins differentiate it from a fracture.
- Stress injuries – the metatarsal is the commonest site for stress fractures, also known as March or fatigue fractures. There may be no evidence of acute trauma, and they can therefore be overlooked. These injuries result from repeated or continuous stress such as walking or running[9,10]. They usually occur in the neck or shaft of the second or third metatarsal and appear as hairline fractures with no displacement. They are usually detected once the callus starts to form 7–14 days post injury. A radioisotope scan or magnetic resonance imaging (MRI) may be necessary to confirm the presence of a stress injury[11].

Fractured phalanges

The first or great toe (Figure 8.6) is most often involved in injuries due to its prominence. Different mechanisms of injury, usually a crush injury from a heavy object or a 'stubbing' injury[12], result in different types of fracture. Crush injuries result in a comminuted fracture of the phalanx; however, the alignment tends to be preserved. Oblique fractures are seen when a toe is caught or 'stubbed' and a chip fracture of the dorsal articular surface follows a hyperflexion injury.

Phalangeal fractures are sometimes associated with damage to the surface of the skin and underlying soft tissue and as such may be extremely painful. This may result in infection, particularly in the immature skeleton. Here, an osteomyelitis or an associated Salter–Harris I injury of the distal phalanx may be seen with nail-bed injuries.

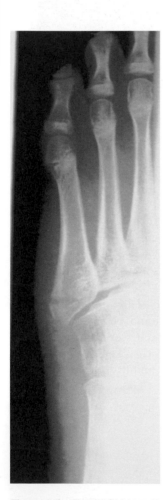

Figure 8.5 Fractured base of the fifth metatarsal – this is usually horizontal or oblique in nature. Apophyseal lines, which are vertical in nature, are often mistaken for fractures along this vector.

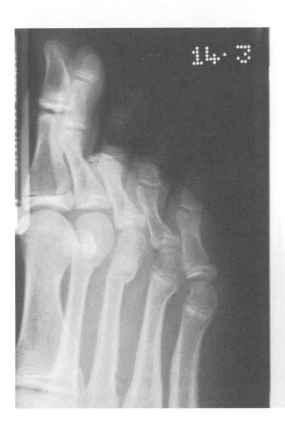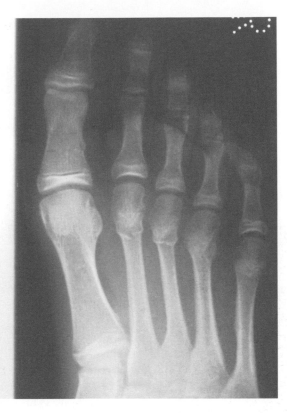

Figure 8.6 Fracture of the proximal phalanx of the hallux. What other fractures are present?

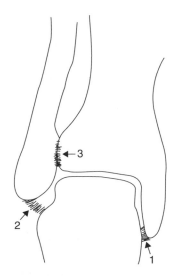

Figure 8.7 The ankle joint as a ring structure:
1 – medical collateral ligament
2 – lateral collateral ligament
3 – interosseous ligament

Remember, whenever a fracture is described, it is important to state whether the fracture extends through the joint margins.

Ankle injuries

The ankle joint is basically a ring structure (Figure 8.7) consisting of the distal tibia, fibula and talus, connected by the following three main groups of ligaments:

Self-test answer

A lucency between the middle and proximal thirds of the proximal phalanx of the right great toe is noted, combined with disruption of the lateral cortex suggesting a fracture is present. Note also the second and third metatarsal neck fractures, and a fracture of the epiphysis of the fourth metatarsal.

Eight

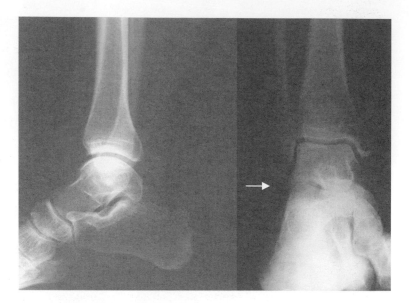

Figure 8.8 The normal ankle.

- medial collateral ligament;
- lateral collateral ligament;
- interosseous ligament.

The ankle (Figure 8.8) is a hinge joint between a mortise that is formed by the lateral and medial malleoli, the distal end of the tibia and the body of the talus. The joint capsule, which fits closely around the articular surfaces, is weak both anteriorly and medially adjacent to the collateral ligaments. The main movements at the ankle joint are plantar- and dorsi-flexion. When the ankle is in plantar-flexion there may be some side-to-side movement as the joint is lax. However, in dorsi-flexion the body of the talus becomes firmly wedged between the malleoli as it is slightly wider anteriorly. These features result in specific injury patterns following certain force vectors. On the mortise (antero-posterior) view check for:

- a uniform joint space; (The width of the joint spaces should be <4 mm medially and 5 mm laterally (superior talar space), otherwise suspect talar tilt. The distance between the tibia and fibula should be <5 mm).
- a smooth talar dome with no apparent defects;
- soft tissue swelling[13];
- avulsion fracture of the tips of the malleoli.

Self-test answer

Essential for correct viewing of the ankle are a clear mortise projection and a lateral projection with superimposition of the talar articular surfaces. In this example an os sub fibulare is present as a round, corticated deposit beneath the tip of the distal fibula (arrow). The base of the fifth metatarsal should also be visible on the lateral projection.

On the lateral view check for:

- the malleoli (the lateral extends more inferiorly than the medial);
- posterior tibia;
- calcaneum;
- base of the fifth metatarsal.

Injuries to the ankle joint may be caused by several different mechanisms and may involve soft tissues alone. The injuries are as follows:

- inversion injuries (supination-adduction);
- eversion injuries (supination-abduction);
- eversion injuries (pronation-external rotation);
- vertical compression injuries.

Fractures may be seen on one view only, and if one fracture is noted it is important to look for a second or for widening of the joint space, which indicates a ligamentous injury. The joint spaces may appear normal despite severe ligament damage. If one side of the joint space appears widened there is likely to be an associated fracture.

Salter–Harris fractures are also common in the immature ankle joint and the less frequently occurring types III and IV are shown in Figure 8.9. SH I of the fibula may be difficult to detect. If epiphysis is angled and accompanied by soft issue swelling then an SH I should be suspected.

Inversion injuries (supination-adduction)

First the lateral ankle structures are affected by avulsive forces. This is followed by stress on the medial structures caused by impactive forces from a secondary talar shift. This may lead to:

- fracture of base of fifth metatarsal
- transverse/oblique fracture of the lateral malleolus in which the tibio-fibular ligaments remain intact;
- oblique fracture of the medial malleolus with or without an associated fracture of the posterior malleolus;
- possible sprain or rupture of the lateral collateral ligament.

An oblique midshaft tibia fracture is seen in Figure 8.10.

An avulsion injury with fractured medial malleolus is seen in Figure 8.11.

Eversion injuries (supination-abduction)

The medial structures of the ankle are subject to avulsive forces, with impaction of the lateral structures (by the talus) (Figure 8.12). This may lead to:

- transverse fractures of the medial malleolus;
- oblique fractures of the lateral malleolus;
- lateral subluxation of the talus;

Eight

(a)

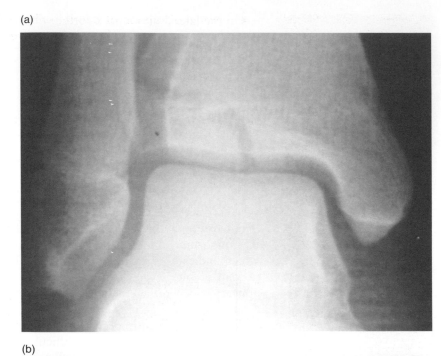

(b)

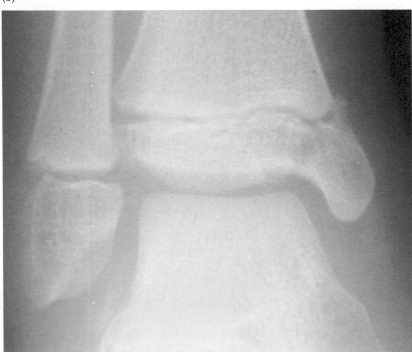

Figure 8.9 The Salter–Harris (a) III and (b) IV injuries.

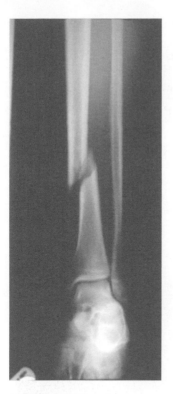

Figure 8.10 An oblique fracture of the tibia.

- partial disruption of the tibio-fibular ligament;
- sprain or rupture of the deltoid ligament.

Pott's fracture

This injury is defined as a fractured fibula above an intact tibio-fibular ligament. There are three degrees of Pott's fracture.

- First – torsional spiral fracture of the lateral malleolus.
- Second – following the spiral fracture, the medial collateral ligament is avulsed and there may be an avulsion fracture of the medial malleolus.
- Third – these are then followed by the posterior margin of the distal tibia being sheared off against the talus as the tibia is carried forward.

For example, a footballer catches his foot in a pothole. The foot is held rigidly in the hole but his body and tibia internally rotate. As the joint space widens the tibia undergoes forward dislocation on the talus, causing the calcaneum to become more prominent – a feature of this injury (Figure 8.13).

Eversion injuries (pronation-external rotation)

The foot is pronated and externally rotated; the anterior and/or posterior tibio-fibular ligaments are torn. These injuries can cause:

Eight

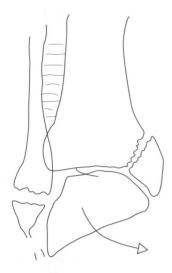

Figure 8.11 Fracture patterns noted following inversion injury. Note the 'pull-off' avulsion of the distal fibula and 'push-off' tibial malleolar fractures.

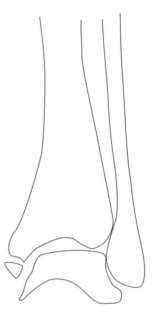

Figure 8.12 Avulsion of the medial malleolus following eversion.

Eight

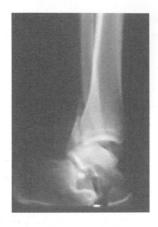

Figure 8.13 Posterior tibial lip fracture – note how the tibia has subluxed anteriorly following loss of structural support.

- avulsion fracture of the anterior tibial tubercle (Tillaux–Chaput fracture);
- avulsion of the posterior tibial tubercle (Volkmann's fracture);
- fibular fracture which is higher than the ankle joint;
- Maissonneuve fracture – fracture of the medial or posterior malleolus and widening of the joint space of the ankle (Figure 8.14), and associated fracture of fibular neck caused by forces transmitted up the interosseous membrane;
- lateral instability due to a tear of the interosseous membrane;
- tear of the tibio-fibular ligament.

(a)   (b)

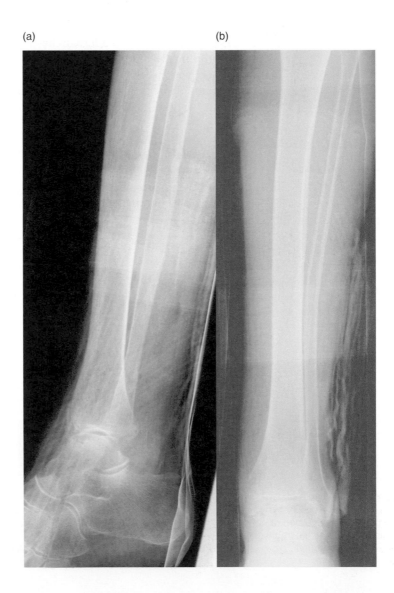

Figure 8.14 Maissonneuve fracture. A fracture of the distal talus (medial and posterior malleolus) is combined with ligamentous disruption causing some talar shift. The immobilisation makes visualisation problematic, but note the bowing of the fibula, with a fracture in the proximal half of the shaft, characteristic of a Maissonneuve fracture.

An oblique fracture of the distal third of the fibula indicates that both the distal tibio-fibular ligaments and the interosseous membrane are disrupted to the level of the fracture.

Vertical compression injuries

These occur following transmission of excessive force through the talus into the distal tibial plafond. This results in the Pilon or 'pestle and mortar' pattern of injury that leads to an intra-articular T- or Y-shaped fracture of the distal tibia. If the foot is dorsi-flexed during the injury, the fracture line tends to be anterior. Identification of the number and size of the fragments is important as this influences the likelihood of surgical intervention and joint stability when more than 30% of the joint surface is involved[14].

Toddler's fracture (Figure 8.15)

This is an oblique or spiral fracture of the tibial shaft, and there is minimal if any displacement. The fracture may be seen only on one view

(a)

(b)

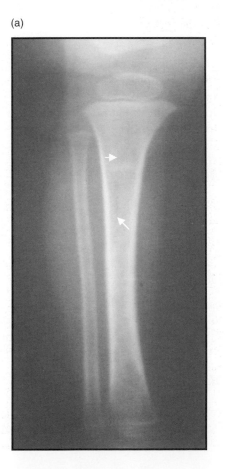
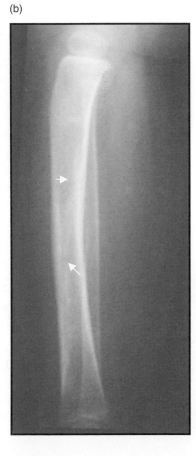

Figure 8.15   (a,b) Toddler's (oblique) fracture of the tibia. The arrows show the direction of the fracture which may be evident as only minimal lucent line.

and is not always apparent on first presentation. Follow-up films may demonstrate a periosteal reaction indicating the presence of a fracture. This fracture is common in infants between the ages of one and three years, and is caused by the child falling with the leg twisted under the body.

Knee injuries

The anatomy of the knee is complex. The distal femoral condyles, proximal tibial plateau and patella are the main osseous structures of the knee. Only 6% of patients with knee trauma actually sustain a fracture. If referral protocols are used to aid decision making when requesting knee radiographs, the number of unnecessary examinations being undertaken may be reduced[15,16]. Two different protocols have been devised and may be used clinically to aid evaluation.

Ottawa knee rules

Criteria for selection of patients who should undergo plain film examination of the knee.

- Age 55 years or older.
- Tenderness at head of fibula.
- Isolated tenderness of patella.
- Inability to flex knee to 90 degrees.
- Inability to walk four weight-bearing steps immediately after the injury and in the A&E department.

Pittsburgh decision rules

- Blunt trauma or fall as the mechanism of injury *plus* either of the following:

- Age younger than 12 years or older than 50 years.
- Inability to walk four weight-bearing steps in the A&E department.

Research has shown that, although there is good sensitivity between the two rules, specificity may not be very high in certain injuries[17]. Fractures can occur in the femoral condyles, the tibial plateau or patella.

Distal femur fractures

Supracondylar fractures tend to occur just proximal to the area where the medial and lateral cortices extend out to the condyles. They are usually transverse, although the condyles can be separated by a vertical fracture, forming a T-shaped fracture. Most supracondylar fractures have a good prognosis and reunite without any complications.

Condylar fractures of the femur are rare and are caused by direct trauma including road traffic accidents. They can range from a crack with no displacement to complete separation with severe displacement (usually posterior). In the young, the associated soft tissue damage can be severe due to the level of force required to cause the fracture.

Patellar fractures

Fractures of the patella may be caused by either a direct force that causes a comminuted or crack fracture, or a sudden explosive contraction of the quadriceps muscle, causing a transverse fracture. Sixty per cent are transverse, through the mid-portion[18]. If a suspected fracture is not clearly demonstrated on the antero-posterior (AP) and lateral views an oblique or skyline (infero-superior) projection may be necessary.

Note: A bipartite or multipartite patella (Figure 8.16) may be confused with a fracture. There are, however, several distinguishing signs.

- The margins of the fragments are smooth.
- The abnormality is often present in the opposite knee.
- The most common site is the supero-lateral corner of the patella, which is a rare site for fractures to occur.

Proximal tibial fractures

Tibial plateau fractures mainly occur in the lateral condyle, as in the case of a pedestrian being hit by the bumper of a car on the lateral border of the knee. They are often associated with damage to the medial collateral ligament and/or the cruciate ligaments. Less commonly, fractures may occur in the medial condyle alone or occasionally in both condyles together.

Impacted fractures of the tibial plateau may be difficult to detect, appearing as a sclerotic line in the condyle. In these circumstances an oblique view may be useful for confirming the diagnosis. The fractures are of three types.

- Comminuted compression fracture – this is most common. The lateral tibial condyle is crushed by the impact of the femoral condyle, causing fragmentation (Figure 8.17).
- Depressed – this is less common. The articular surface of the lateral condyle is depressed but does not fragment.
- Oblique shearing – this is least common. A large section of the lateral condyle is sheared off through an oblique fracture.

On a normal AP projection of the knee, the femoral condyles and upper tibia are in alignment. Where the tibial plateau is fractured, the

Eight

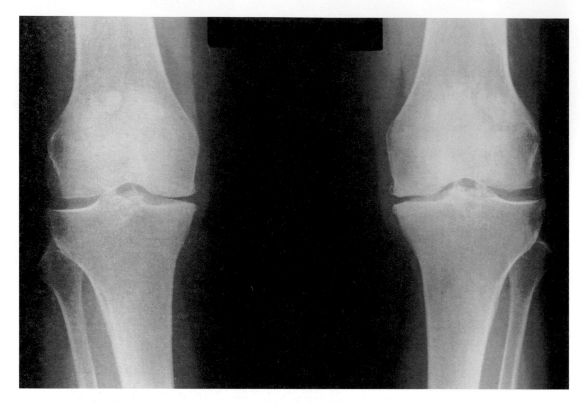

Figure 8.16   The multipartite patella.

margin of the tibia is often displaced, causing a step at the knee joint. If a perpendicular line is drawn at the lateral margin of the femur, no more than 5 mm of the adjacent tibial margin should be beyond it. If this occurs a lateral tibial plateau fracture should be suspected (Figure 8.18).

Most knee fractures are easily detected but there are occasions when an intra-articular fracture is only discovered on a horizontal beam lateral radiograph, when a fat–fluid level is demonstrated in the supra-patellar bursa (Figures 8.19 and 8.20). The joint effusion may contain fat from the bone marrow released through the fracture site. The fat lies on top of the blood, creating a fat–fluid level known as a lipohaemarthrosis. This indicates an intra-articular fracture even when one cannot clearly be visualised[19].

Self-test answer

Remember, the bipartite patella may be confused with a fracture from the supero-lateral corner of the knee-cap. However, its rounded appearance and apparent association with the main bone allows the viewer to be certain an injury has not occurred.

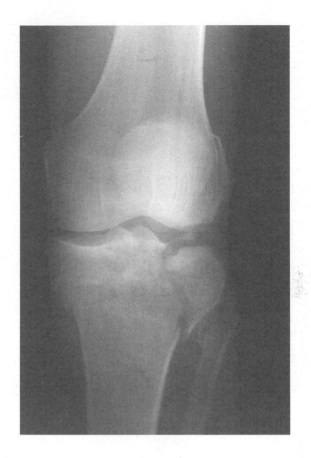

Eight

Figure 8.17 A comminuted fracture of the tibial plateau.

Avulsion of the tibial spine (Figure 8.21)

This is rare and is caused by the cruciate ligament pulling off a fragment of bone from the intercondylar ridge of the tibia. An alternative cause is a fall from a bicycle (often a young child) to land on the flexed knee,

Self-test answer

In the (left) tibia there is an intra-articular fracture line running infero-laterally from the lateral tibial spine, communicating with a horizontal fracture slightly inferior to the epiphyseal scar. This has led to depression and lateral shift of this free portion of the tibial plateau by several millimetres. A further oblique fracture line is seen travelling infero-laterally from the horizontal fracture identified above to the lateral cortex. At least two bone fragments are seen in the joint space of the knee. There is a horizontal fracture of the neck of the left fibula.

Eight

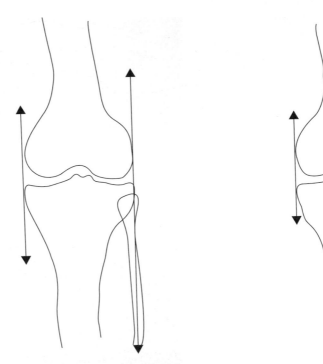

Figure 8.18 Assessment of the frontal projection of the tibia in suspected fractures of the tibial plateau should take account of the alignment of the medial and lateral borders of femur with the tibia. Any discrepancy would be suggestive of medial or lateral slip of the fracture fragment.

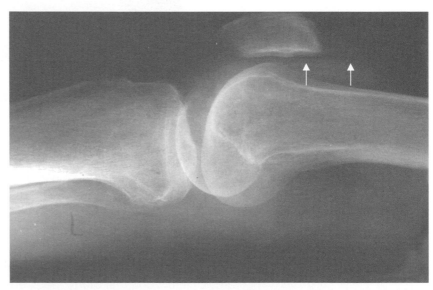

Figure 8.19 The lipohaemarthrosis (arrows) as an indicator of subtle intra-articular fracture.

thus directing a shearing force along the tibial plateau, resulting in fracture along the base of the tibial spine.

Pellegrini–Steida disease

Occasionally an incomplete avulsion of the medial collateral ligament of the medial condyle of the femur causes ossification in the haematoma

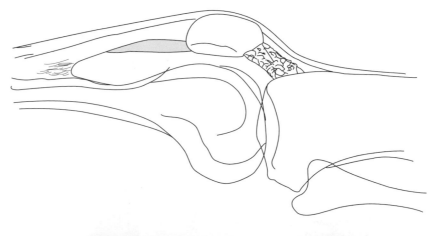

Figure 8.20 The lipohaemarthrosis revealed diagrammatically. Lighter, radiolucent fat sits on top of blood in the suprapatellar region, both of which have leaked from an intra-articular bone fracture that may not be apparent on the images produced.

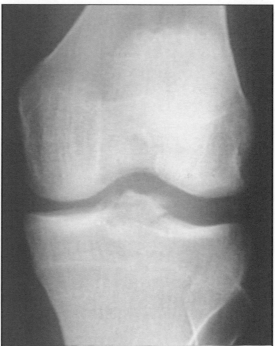

Figure 8.21 Tibial spine avulsion.

that forms between the ligament and the femoral condyle, known as Pellegrini–Steida disease (Figure 8.22).

Segond fracture (Figure 8.23)

Rotation at the knee causes tensing of the ilio-tibial band, which inserts at Gurdy's tubercle on the lateral side of the proximal tibia above the fibular head[20]. The image should be scrutinised carefully and the joint width assessed for congruence as these injuries indicate severe rotation that could have associated internal damage.

Eight

(a) (b)

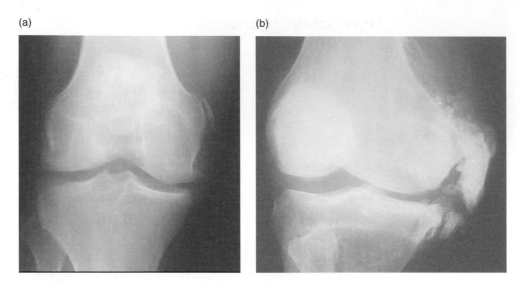

Figure 8.22 The Pellegrini–Steida lesion in various stages of development. (a) Minor/early changes and (b) chronic or long-standing disease.

(a) (b)

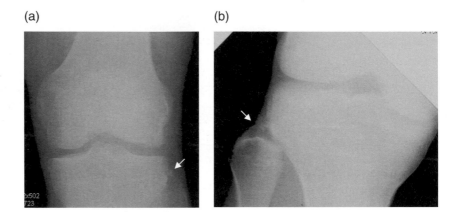

Figure 8.23 (a,b) The Segond fracture displayed via an AP and oblique projection (arrows).

Dislocation

Dislocation of the knee is extremely rare, and serious complications include injury to the popliteal artery or one of the main nerve routes. Less serious are late-onset osteoarthritis, instability of the joint and restricted movements. Lateral dislocation of the patella may result from an acute injury while the knee is in flexion or is semi-flexed. Occasionally, recurrent or habitual dislocation of the patella caused by shortening of the quadriceps muscle may occur, more commonly in young girls around the age of 13–18 years (recurrent) or in early childhood (habitual).

Ligamentous injuries

Plain radiographs may be useful in the initial diagnosis of ligamentous injuries; however, they are not necessarily the technique of choice. MRI may be more appropriate for determining and classifying the extent of the injury.

Anterior cruciate ligament

Rupture of this ligament is a serious injury. Three important radiographic signs may be present:

- avulsion of the intercondylar tubercle;
- anterior displacement of the tibia in relation to the femur;
- the avulsion of a small sliver of bone from the proximal lateral tibia where the capsule inserts – the lateral capsular sign. There may be similarities with the Segond pattern described above[21].

Injuries may be caused by hyperextension or valgus force combined with external rotation of the tibia relative to the femur.

Posterior cruciate ligament

These are rare due to the strength of this ligament. The usual mechanism of injury is direct trauma to the anterior tibia, e.g. 'dashboard' injury. The radiographic sign is avulsion of the ligament on the posterior aspect of the tibia or at the point of insertion of the ligament at the medial femoral condyle.

Collateral ligaments

The radiographic sign of medial collateral ligament injury is widening of the medial joint space, coupled with a possible fractured lateral tibial plateau. Conversely, damage to the lateral collateral ligament may be demonstrated by widening of the lateral joint space and a medial tibial plateau fracture.

Proximal femur injuries

A fractured neck of femur is the most frequent cause of traumatic death over the age of 75 years. There is a high incidence in elderly women due to falls, frailty and osteoporosis, with a 20% risk of a fractured femur

Eight

in a 90-year-old woman compared with a 10% risk in a 90-year-old man[3,22]. Fractures are unusual in young adults, who are more likely to sustain fractures of the acetabulum or dislocations of the hip.

Fractures of the femoral neck and intertrochanteric region

The main vascular supply is from the medial and lateral circumflex arteries that form a ring around the base of the femoral neck. They are vulnerable to injury if the neck of femur is fractured and may predispose to avascularity and subsequent avascular necrosis of the femoral head and neck. Important points about injuries of these areas include:

- 63% involve the femoral neck – predominantly in women;
- 37% involve the intertrochanteric region – particulary in patients with osteoarthritis, a slightly greater female to male ratio;
- osteoporosis is a very important factor and the more advanced the condition the more likely it is a fracture may occur. It has been shown that trabecular sub-clinical fractures occur in the femoral neck in women with osteoporosis – trabecular fragility fractures;
- in some elderly patients fractures occur without trauma – insufficiency fractures;
- in young people, fractures of the femoral shaft are much more likely.

Classification of femoral neck fractures

General classification of hip fractures is given in Table 8.1. The typical clinical findings of femoral neck fractures are shortening of the affected side and external rotation of the femoral neck. However, if there is no displacement of the fracture fragments, then there will be no deformity – only pain and an inability to bear weight. Two indicators are used:

(1)   the renowned smoothly curving Shenton's line (Figure 8.24) that arcs from the lesser trochanter medially to follow the line formed by the inferior surface of the superior pubic ramus;
(2)   the lines of the primary trabecular pattern, which help to indicate the presence of a fracture through disruption or apparent crowding due to impaction.

The subsequent healing of a fracture may also be influenced by whether the fracture is:

1.   **Intracapsular** – the main determinant of healing is the vascular supply because the major vessels cross the femoral neck on the lateral aspect (Figure 8.25). The likelihood of avascular necrosis (AVN) increases with the degree of displacement of the bone fragments. The radiographic appearances of AVN may be delayed for up to three years, or as long as five years following internal fixation of displaced fractures.

Eight

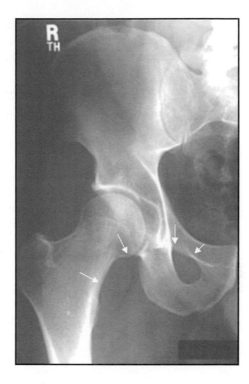

Figure 8.24 Shenton's line.

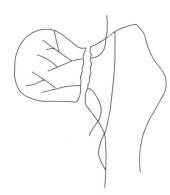

Figure 8.25 The intra-capsular hip fracture demonstrating loss of blood supply to the femoral head raising the possible sequel of avascular necrosis.

Table 8.1 General classification of hip fractures, adapted from Heller and Fink (2000).

Fracture type	Location	Comments
Capital (femoral head)	Intra-capsular	Usually associated with hip dislocation. Caused by impaction of head on acetabular rim. Compression fractures more common than shearing fractures.
Femoral neck	Intra-capsular	May occur following significant injury, or spontaneously in osteoporotic women and athletes (stress fracture). More common than intertrochanteric fractures. 3 types: 1. subcapital: junction of femoral head and neck (most common location, see Garden classification) 2. midcervical: middle of femoral neck, often occur in children following severe trauma 3. basocervical: base of neck, rare in trauma, mainly pathological or stress fracture
Trochanteric	Extra-capsular	Occur following higher forces than femoral neck. Mainly elderly, with males/female equally affected. Heal better than neck fractures due to better vascularisation. 3 types: 1. intertrochanteric: fractures between greater and lesser trochanter (similar to basocervical appearance) 2. subtrochanteric: within 5 cm below lesser trochanter 3. avulsion of the trochanters: lesser more commonly affected in children (contraction of iliopsoas muscle), greater more common in adults (direct injury)

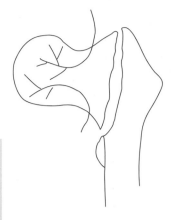

Figure 8.26 An extra-capsular (basicervical) fracture of the hip without damage to the femoral head blood supply.

2. **Extracapsular** – the intertrochanteric region is better supplied with blood vessels, therefore the prognosis for healing is better and there is less likelihood of AVN (Figure 8.26).

Intertrochanteric fractures (Figure 8.27)

These are usually comminuted fractures, and as the degree of comminution increases the greater the degree of instability. Avulsion fractures of the trochanters may occur in the elderly as a result of falls. They are often comminuted but rarely displaced and AVN is infrequent[24]. Avulsion fractures of the lesser trochanter usually occur in children or adolescents as the apophysis is avulsed by the iliopsoas. In adults this

Self-test answer

There is an evident flattening of Shenton's line of the right hip in comparison with the left. Closer evaluation reveals an intertrochanteric fracture line and loss of continuity between the femoral neck and shaft typical of this type of injury.

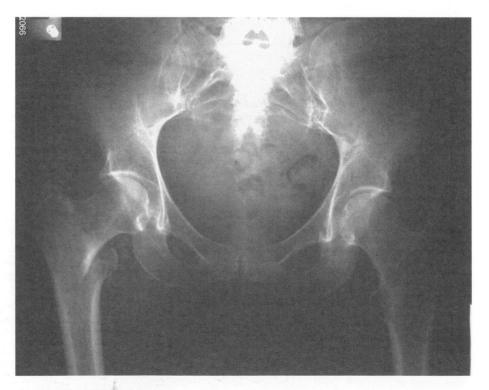

Figure 8.27 The intertrochanteric fracture.

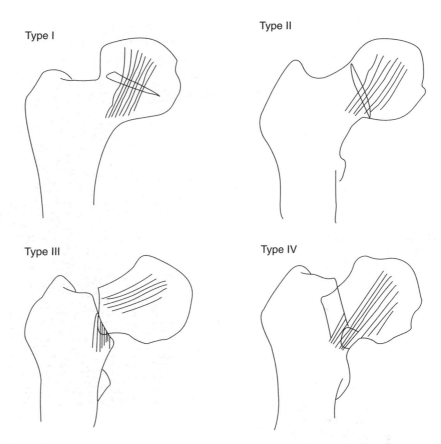

Type I

Type II

Type III

Type IV

Figure 8.28 The Garden classification of hip fractures. With increasing number the stability of the injury reduces. Adapted from Evans and McGrory (2004).

Table 8.2 Garden classification of femoral hip fractures.

Type	Description
Type I	Valgus impaction of the femoral head
Type II	Complete but non-displaced fracture
Type III	Varus displacement of the femoral head
Type IV	Complete loss of continuity between both fragments

injury raises suspicion of an underlying abnormality such as metastatic disease.

Garden classification

The Garden classification describes the final positions and angles of the various fractures of the neck of femur. As with most systems the higher the number in the sequence of the injury, the greater the likelihood of complications. As mentioned earlier, the greater the displacement of fracture components, the greater the chance of AVN. Figures 8.28 and 8.29 and Table 8.2 give an overview of the classification.

Eight

(a) Type I

(b) Type II

(c) Type III

(d) Type IV

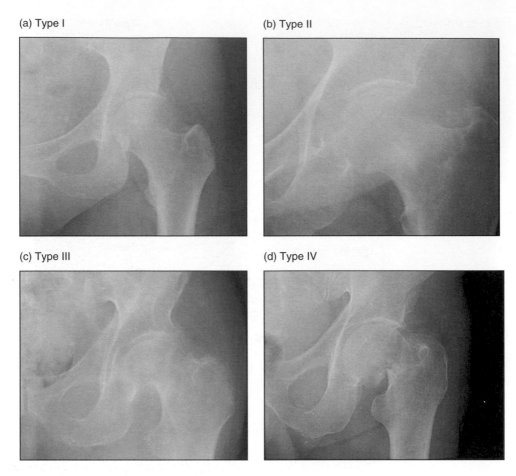

Figure 8.29   The Garden classification of hip fractures.

Dislocation and fracture-dislocation of the hip

Relatively rare, these are usually a result of a road traffic accident[26]; commonest is posterior dislocation (90%) which follows anterior force to the flexed knee to displace the femoral head posteriorly. Typically this results from a dashboard impact. Fractures of the femoral shaft may be associated with posterior dislocations and if femur projections are inadequate the diagnosis may be missed. Usually a posterior acetabular lip fracture is evident. The possibility of associated fractures of the femoral head should also be considered. There are two types.

- **Shear** – a slice of the femoral head becomes detached due to the impact of the femur on the posterior acetabular margin.
- **Compression** – involves the anterior aspect of the femoral head. Computed tomography (CT) may assist in confirming the diagnosis.

Less common are anterior dislocations (Figure 8.30), which result from abduction and external rotation. The femoral head may come to rest beneath

Eight

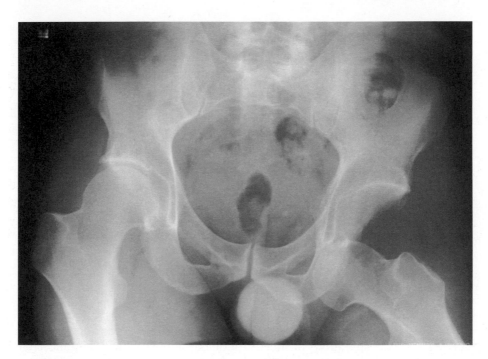

Figure 8.30 Anterior hip dislocation.

the iliac spine or pubis. They can be associated with fractures of the femoral head. Central dislocations occur when the head of the femur is forced through the acetabulum into the pelvis. The acetabulum is comminuted.

Stress and insufficiency fractures of the femoral neck

These tend to occur in athletes, patients with abnormal bone such as in rheumatoid arthritis, and very occasionally in the elderly. Stress fractures may not always be seen on plain films and isotope imaging or CT follow-up may be indicated[27].

Paediatric considerations

Fractures of the hip are rare in children. The most common cause of hip pain in children is irritable hip (transient synovitis), which is thought to be of viral aetiology. Other, more serious, possibilities to consider are:

Self-test answer

The head of the left femur lies below the tear-drop of the acetabulum, having moved infero-medially. This would be indicative of an anterior hip dislocation.

Eight

- a slipped upper femoral epiphysis, where the epiphysis slips posteriorly and medially. This is more common in boys and rarely occurs in children under the age of eight years;
- Perthes' disease (osteochondritis of the femoral head), again more common in boys.

Slipped upper femoral epiphysis

This is one of the most significant hip disorders of adolescence. It is a progressive disorder that requires early diagnosis and intervention. The femoral head 'slips' posteriorly and into varus. It tends to occur in obese skeletally immature children, with a male to female ratio of 3 : 1. Twenty per cent of cases are bilateral and approximately 5% have a family history[26]. Patients usually present with a gradual onset of either hip or knee pain, although sudden onset of pain following exercise may also occur.

Radiologically, the diagnosis may be difficult. On an AP projection the epiphyseal plate appears widened with less distinct margins, and the epiphysis appears shorter. A 'frog lateral' can aid the diagnosis. Complications include AVN due to impaired blood supply. **Trethowan's sign** is a positive indicator of a slipped femoral epiphysis (Figure 8.31). On the AP projection of the hip, a line drawn along the superior surface of the neck of the femur should pass through the femoral head. If the line passes superiorly to the femoral head then the epiphysis has slipped.

Perthes' disease

It may appear unusual to include this here. However, trauma or chronic stress is thought to be the underlying aetiology, and it is seen between 2 and 14 years with a peak between 4 and 9 years. Boys are affected four times more frequently than girls[28] but the latter have an earlier age of onset and a worse prognosis. It is bilateral in 10% of cases. There is no evidence of increased familial incidence, but parents of affected children are often elderly. Affected children may show skeletal growth retardation and associated congenital abnormalities. Symptoms are usually long-standing with a limp, pain and limited motion at the hip. Fixed flexion and adduction may result with shortening and muscle wasting.

Radiologically, the earliest sign is that of a joint effusion with resultant widening of the joint space. The femoral head may be displaced laterally 2–5 mm. A subchondral fracture may be seen on the lateral radiograph as a radiolucent crescent on the postero-medial aspect of the femoral head (Figure 8.32). There is reduction in size of the ossification nucleus of the epiphysis due to growth retardation. The epiphyseal centre becomes flattened, fragmented and dense. Lytic areas may be seen in the metaphysis; these represent fibrous tissue or cartilage which has infiltrated this area. See also Figure 6.42 on p. 103.

Eight

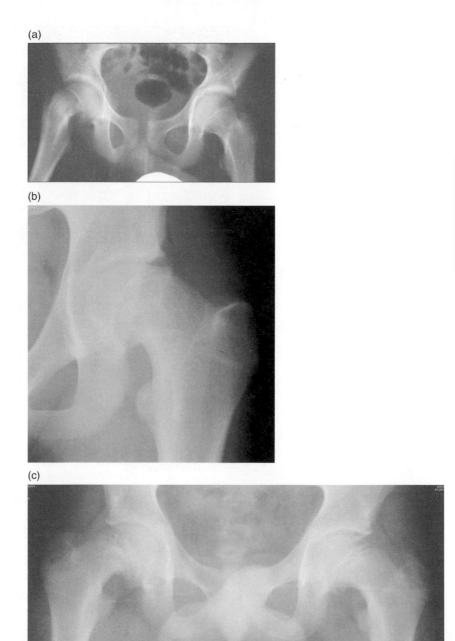

(a)

(b)

(c)

Figure 8.31 (a,b) Slipped upper femoral epiphysis. (c) Bilateral slipped epiphyses.

Self-test answer (a,b)

Trethowan's test is positive showing slipping of the left upper femoral epiphysis.

Eight

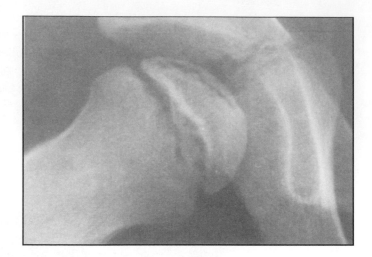

Figure 8.32
Legg–Calvé–Perthes disease
of the femoral head. Note the
subchondral lucency
characteristic of early necrosis.

Table 8.3   Ossification dates for the lower limb.

Bone	Primary/ secondary	Site	Appearance	Fuses
Pelvis	1	Ilium		
		Ischium		
		Pubis		16th/18th year
	2	Iliac crest	13th year	20th/25th year
		AIIS	13th year	16th/18th year
Femur	1	Shaft	7th week IU	
	2	Head	6 months	
		Greater trochanter	4th year	With shaft
		Lesser trochanter	13th/14th year	at puberty
		Lower end	9th month IU	
Patella	1		3rd/6th year	
Tibia	1	Shaft	7th week IU	
	2	Upper end	Birth	
		Lower end	1st year	17th/18th year
Fibula	1	Shaft	8th week IU	
	2	Upper end	4th/5th year	
		Lower end	1st year	15/17th year
Tarsals	1	Calcaneum	6th month IU	
		Talus	7th month IU	
		Cuboid	9th month IU	
		Lateral cuneiform	1st year	
		Medial cuneiform	3rd year	
		Int cuneiform	4th year	
		Navicular	4th year	
	2	Post-calceneum	6th/8th year	14th/16th year
Metatarsals	1	Shaft	9th/10th	
	2	Head (base of first)	3rd/4th year	17th/20th year
Phalanges	1	Shaft	9th/16th week IU	
			2nd/8th year	18th year

AIIS, anterior inferior iliac spine; IU, *in utero*.

Complications

Patients who have a poor result following treatment of the disease are left with a stable hip which has been converted from a ball and socket joint to a saddle joint; however, they are capable of a relatively free amount of movement within the range of the modified point. Severe secondary degenerative joint disease follows prematurely.

A final thought . . .

This chapter has presented a fairly brief overview of the radiographic pattern of injuries to the lower limb. Injuries are seen as a result of bone immaturity; however, misinterpretation arising from the extent of epiphyseal fusion is relatively common. Table 8.3 summarises the dates of fusion of ossification centres in the lower limb which are worth bearing in mind when reviewing plain film images of the traumatised skeleton.

References

1 Prokuski, L.J. and Saltzman, C.L. (1997) Challenging fractures of the foot and ankle. *Radiologic Clinics of North America* **35**(3), 655–70.
2 Loomer, R., Fisher, C., Lloyd-Smith R., *et al.* (1993) Osteochondral lesions of the talus. *American Journal of Sports Medicine* **21**(1), 13–19.
3 Manaster, B.J. (1997) *Handbooks in Radiology: Skeletal Radiology.* Mosby, London.
4 Raby, N., Berman, L. and de Lacey, G. (1995) *Accident and Emergency Radiology: A Survival Guide.* WB Saunders, London.
5 Felder-Johnson, K.L., Murdoch, D.P. and McGanity, P. (1995) Lisfranc's fracture. A literature review and case presentations of tarsometatarsal joint injuries. Dislocation. *Clinics in Podiatric Medicine and Surgery* **12**(4), 565–602.
6 Brown, D.D. and Gumbs, R.V. (1991) Lisfranc fracture-dislocation: report of two cases. *Journal of the National Medical Association* **83**(4), 366–9.
7 Urteaga, A.J. and Lynch, M. (1995) Fractures of the central metatarsals. *Clinics in Podiatric Medicine and Surgery* **12**(4), 759–72.
8 Strayer, S.M., Reece, S.G. and Patrizzi, M.J. (1999) Fractures of the proximal fifth metatarsal. *American Family Physician* **59**(9), 216–22.
9 Pester, S. and Smith, C. (1992) Stress fractures in the lower extremities of soldiers in basic training. *Orthopaedic Review* **21**(3), 297–303.
10 Frey, C. (1997) Footwear and stress fractures. *Clinics in Sports Medicine* **16**(2), 249–57.
11 Chowchuen, P. and Resnick, D. (1998) Stress fractures of the metatarsal heads. *Skeletal Radiology* **27**(1), 22–5.

Eight

12   David, H.G. and Freedman, L.S. (1990) Injuries caused by tripping over paving stones: an unappreciated problem. *British Medical Journal* **300**(6727), 784–5.

13   Clark, T.W., Janzen, D.L. and Ho, K. (1995) Detection of radiographically occult ankle fractures following acute trauma: positive predictive value of an ankle effusion. *American Journal of Roentgenology* **164**(5), 1185–9.

14   Raasch, W.G., Larkin, J.J. and Draganich, L.F. (1992) Assessment of the posterior malleolus as a restraint to posterior subluxation of the ankle. *Journal of Bone and Joint Surgery (American Edition)* **74**(8), 1201–06.

15   Stiell, I.G., Wells, G.A., McDowell, I., *et al.* (1995) Use of radiography in acute knee injuries: need for clinical decision rules. *Academic Emergency Medicine* **2**(11), 966–73.

16   Stiell, I.G., Wells, G.A., Hoag, R.H., *et al.* (1997) Implementation of the Ottawa knee rule for the use of radiography in acute knee injuries. Comment in: *Journal of American Medical Association* **278**(23), 2108–09.

17   Richman, P.B., MuCuskey, C.F., Nashed, A., *et al.* (1997) Performance of two clinical decision rules for knee radiography. *Journal of Emergency Medicine* **15**(4), 459–63.

18   Manaster, B.J. and Andrews, C.L. (1994) Fractures and dislocations of the knee and proximal tibia and fibula. *Seminars in Roentgenology* **29**(2), 113–33.

19   Ferguson, J. and Knottenbelt, J.D. (1994) Lipohaemarthrosis in knee trauma: an experience of 907 cases. *Injury* **25**(5), 311–12.

20   Kozin, S.H. and Berlet, A.C. (1992) *Handbook of Common Orthopaedic Fractures*, 2nd edn. Medical Surveillance Inc, Westchester, PA.

21   Davis, D.S. and Post, W.R. (1997) Segond fracture: lateral capsular ligament avulsion. *Journal of Orthopaedic and Sports Physical Therapy* **25**(2), 103–06.

22   Kannus, P., Pakkari, J., Sievanen, H., *et al.* (1996) Epidemiology of hip fractures. *Bone* **18**(1 suppl), 57S–63S.

23   Heller, M. and Fink, A. (2000) *Radiology of Trauma*, Springer–Verlag, Berlin.

24   Baixauli, E.J., Baixauli, F., Jr, Baixauli, F., *et al.* (1999) Avascular necrosis of the femoral head after intertrochanteric fractures [corrected and republished version]. *Journal of Orthopaedic Trauma* **13**(2), 134–7.

25   Evans, P.J. and McGrory, B.J. (2004) Fractures of the Proximal Femur, *Orthopaedic Associates of Portland*, www.orthoassociates.com/hipfx.htm

26   Nikolic, V., Ruszkowski, I., Elabjer, E., *et al.* (1995) Biomechanical features of axial injuries to the lower limbs and to the pelvic ring by motor car collisions. *Acta Medica Croatica* **49**(1), 21–8.

27   Deutch, A.L., Coerl, M.N. and Mink, J.H. (1997) Imaging of stress injuries to bone. Radiography, scintigraphy and MR imaging. *Clinics in Sports Medicine* **16**(2), 275–90.

28   Burnett, S., Taylor, A. and Watson, M. (2000) *A–Z of Orthopaedic Radiology*. WB Saunders, London.

Eight

9

The Spine

Introduction

This chapter explains how the spine works as a mechanical unit to allow the image reader to interpret the patterns that may be presented. It discusses the anatomy, pathomechanics and the influence of some pathologies and describes likely presentations in both children and adults. Soft tissue injury, dislocation and fracture patterns will also be discussed, and normal variations, image artefacts and the effects of sub-optimal imaging examined.

In reviewing vertebral anatomy, each individual vertebra has two essential components:

- vertebral body;
- neural arch.

These articulate with the vertebra above and below to form the spinal column, operating in conjunction with associated soft tissues. Table 9.1 summarises the components of the spine. The ligaments are illustrated in Figure 9.1.

Spinal mechanics

Movement and therefore injury to the spine are based on a three-column concept developed by Denis in 1983 (Table 9.2 and Figure 9.2). The middle column effectively communicates with the anterior and posterior columns as a pivot with the latter columns forming the arms of a seesaw. This has resulted in the concept that following trauma if the:

- middle column is intact – spine is stable;
- middle column is disrupted – spine is unstable.

Table 9.1   Components of the spine.

Anterior components	Posterior components
Vertebral body	Pedicles
Intervertebral discs	Facets
Anterior and posterior longitudinal ligaments	Apophyseal joints and capsules
	Laminae
	Spinous process
	Ligaments

Ligamentous components	
Anterior longitudinal	Flavum
Tautly bound to the anterior body and annulus of the disc	Lines the dorsal canal surface and is anchored to the laminae
Posterior longitudinal	Interspinous
Weaker, but bound to the posterior body and disc	Interconnects the spinous processes
	Supraspinous
	Contiguously connects the dorsal tip of the spinous process from occiput to sacrum

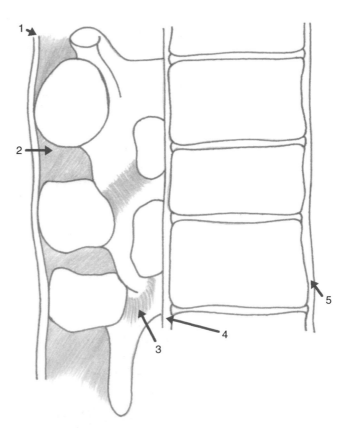

Figure 9.1 Ligaments of the typical vertebrae. Applicable to all typical vertebrae, the ligaments that are seen here are present throughout the vertebral column.

1   Supraspinous ligament
2   Interspinous ligament
3   Apophyseal (facet) joint capsule
4   Posterior longitudinal ligament
5   Anterior longitudinal ligament

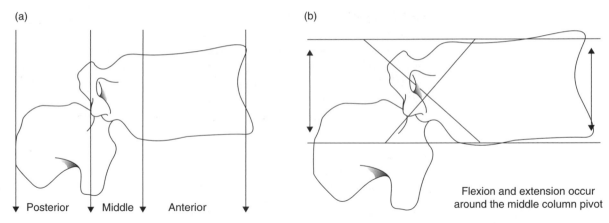

Figure 9.2 (a,b) The three-column model of force transmission. The various columns contain different structures. The anterior consists of the anterior two-thirds of the vertebral body and any ligaments. The middle column is made up of all structures in the posterior third of the vertebral body to the pedicles. The posterior column is from the pedicles to the spinous processes. Injuries to specific parts of the vertebral column around the central fulcrum therefore become apparent.

Table 9.2 Components of the three-column concept.

Column	Components
Anterior	Anterior vertebral body, annulus fibrosus and anterior longitudinal ligament
Middle	Posterior vertebral body, annulus fibrosus and posterior longitudinal ligament
Posterior	Neural arch and adjacent soft tissues

Mechanics of injury

Spinal injuries normally arise from an indirect force generated by moving the head and trunk beyond the limits imposed by vertebral construction. Occasionally direct blows may cause injury. A range of forces combine together in spinal trauma, these include:

- flexion;
- compression;
- extension;
- rotation;
- shearing;
- distraction.

A general rule is that:

- rotational and shearing forces disrupt ligaments;
- compressive forces generate fractures.

Flexion

This is the most common indirect force in injury. Anterior arching of the spine about the middle column pivot creates vertebral body compression and neural arch tension, resulting in anterior body wedging from compression and posterior structure fractures and ligamentous disruption from tension. Maximum force is focused in two main areas.

- When the movement of the head is towards the trunk, force acts between the C4 and C7 cervical bodies.
- In the trunk, flexion causes injuries between T12 and L2 vertebral bodies (see Figures 9.3 and 9.4)

Compression

Compression injuries occur with the spine positioned neutrally with vertical or axial loads being placed on the vertebrae without spinal angulation. Compression occurs in all three columns with the vertebral discs and bodies absorbing the shock. The vertebral end plate bulges, until eventually blood may be squeezed from the cancellous bone. If the pressure rises further a concave vertebral body end plate fracture will result.

A burst fracture will be generated following increasing pressure as a result of disc bulging and eventual explosion into the vertebral body. This generates a sagittally oriented, comminuted fracture whose fragments are displaced sidewards and backwards from the centre of the exploding disc.

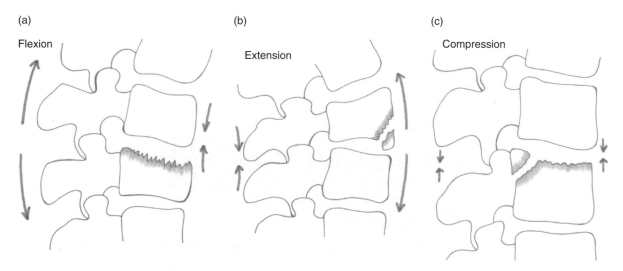

(a) Flexion   (b) Extension   (c) Compression

Figure 9.3   (a–c) Pathomechanics of spinal injury – flexion, compression and extension.

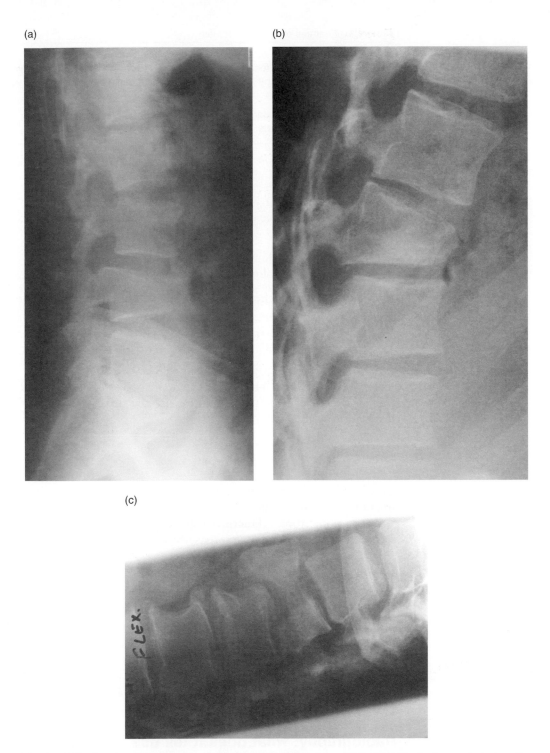

Nine

Figure 9.4 (a–c) Varying degrees of flexion wedging of the lumbar spine. Most disruption is demonstrated on the horizontal ray image (9.4c).

Table 9.3   Features of extension forces.

Anteriorly	Tension of the anterior longitudinal ligament
	Tearing at the intervertebral disc space or vertebral body margin
	Avulsion of the antero-superior or antero-inferior corner of the vertebral body
Posteriorly	Compression may result in fractures of the spinous processes, laminae and facets

Extension

This is the reverse force of flexion about the pivot of the middle column. The result is that:

- the anterior column is placed under tension;
- the posterior column is compressed.

Extension about the head and trunk results in the features noted in Table 9.3.

Rotation

These forces cause interspinous ligament disruption and posterior element fractures. Rotational injuries are the prime cause for fracture-dislocation of the spine.

Shearing

This is the horizontal force applied to one portion of the spine relative to another. It tends to disrupt ligaments, and the force is often combined with rotational forces. Fracture-dislocations of the thoracic and lumbar spine are often seen following these forces.

Distraction

This is the opposite of compression. Momentum and inertia of the head in cervical spine injuries are important. The momentum of the head moving away from the cervical spine is converted into tensile forces. The force direction is dictated by the direction of movement of the head resulting in fractures through the transverse axis of the vertebra.

Figure 9.5 illustrates rotation, shearing and distraction.

Radiography: what does it tell us?

Following spinal trauma, radiographs should provide answers to two questions.

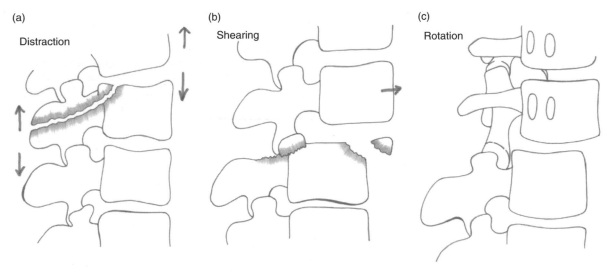

Figure 9.5   (a–c) Pathomechanics of spinal injury – shearing, rotation and distraction.

- Is there a fracture or dislocation?
- Is the injury stable?

The degree of instability depends upon the extent of disruption and relative strength of the remaining intact structures. Soft tissue damage can only be inferred by assessing variations in alignment and distance between bone structures normally anchored by soft tissues. Of particular importance is the widening in disc spaces and spinous processes. This offsets spinal structures anteriorly and posteriorly, respectively. It should be noted that widening of spinous processes also offsets adjacent structures laterally.

Take note:

- The signs of injury evident on the radiograph often underestimate the true extent of damage at the time of trauma.
- Tailoring of the normal antero-posterior (AP) and lateral projections may be necessary – this may include obliques or rarely flexion/extension stress projections under medical supervision. This may be seen as a controversial approach especially in the light of the availability of other imaging modalities (such as computed tomography (CT) and magnetic resonance imaging (MRI)) in cases where neurological change is clinically evident.

Injury classification

It is convenient to consider the spine in three sections.

Table 9.4 The principal categories of injury and their characteristics.

Category	Characteristic
Flexion	Anterior wedge fracture of vertebral body
Extension	Vertebral body is intact or there may be a minimally displaced small avulsion fracture at the antero-superior or inferior margin of the vertebral body
Burst	The vertebral body fracture fragment is forcefully propelled back into the spinal canal.
Distraction	Vertebral body retains normal anterior height but suffers a horizontal fracture of the posterior body/neural arch
Translation – a combination of shearing and rotation	Subluxation or obvious dislocation is revealed by malalignment of neighbouring vertebral bodies axially

(1) Atlanto-axial – includes occipital condyles, C1 and C2.
(2) Cervical spine – C3 to C7.
(3) Thoracolumbar – includes all the thoracic and lumbar vertebrae.

Table 9.4 shows the principal categories of injury and their characteristics.

Injuries of the thoracolumbar spine

- In adults, 60–70% of thoracolumbar spine fractures occur at T12, L1 and L2 with 90% of all fractures being seen between T11 and L4.
- Fractures in the middle or upper thoracic spine are rare in adults but are relatively common in children at T4 and T5 with an associated injury at L2. Often children exhibit contiguous fractures through several vertebrae.
- Twenty per cent of thoracolumbar fractures are seen in association with other skeletal injuries such as the thoracolumbar junction and the calcaneus, or the upper thoracic spine and sternum.

Plain film assessment with a suspicion of fracture

- A paraspinal mass is the indirect finding seen on the antero-posterior projection (often bilaterally but asymmetrically) close to the spine following the formation of a haematoma which lifts the paraspinous ligaments (Figure 9.6) that lie alongside the thoracic spine. This mass may extend beyond the fracture site.
- The paraspinal haematoma in upper thoracic spine fractures forms a pleural cap to mimic the appearance of traumatic aortic dis-

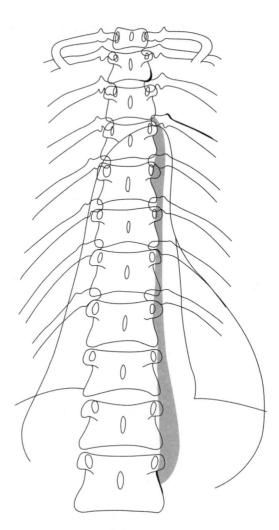

Figure 9.6 The normal paraspinal line. The paraspinous ligaments are usually invisible. However, following trauma they may be elevated by haematoma to become visible alongside the spine, particularly in the thoracic region.

ruption. The viewer should confirm that a dorsal spine fracture is present on the images obtained so patient management does not include angiographic studies.

- When considering the AP projection of the thoracolumbar spine remember:
  - the vertebral body is seen with the posterior elements superimposed on it;
  - pedicles are ovoid;
  - the cortical surfaces of the spinous processes are 'tear-drop' shaped;
  - the adjacent inferior and superior articular facets are well seated within each other;
  - the laminae are displayed as solid bony plates.
- Clues to disruption of the posterior elements on the AP projection include the following:

Nine

- - Transverse fracture or ligamentous disruption posteriorly shows angulation of the superior fracture fragment (or vertebra) so the posterior elements are no longer superimposed on the whole vertebral body. The vertebral body appears empty and the interspinous distance will be increased. In fractures a transverse line through the spinous processes will show fragment separation.
  - Loss of continuity in the spinous process tear-shaped cortex or the ovoid appearance of the pedicle with an accompanying transverse fracture line through the articular processes or laminae.
- Paraspinous haematoma and abrupt angulation in vertebral alignment are diagnostic of middle to lower thoracic spine fractures/dislocations.
- Clues to injury visualised on the lateral thoracolumbar spine projections include:
  - loss of vertebral body height following vertebral wedging;
  - fanning of the spinous processes;
  - loss of joint congruence between the intervertebral facet joint relations;
  - stepping anteriorly or posteriorly of the vertical alignment of the vertebral structures. This could be the anterior or posterior edges of the vertebral bodies or loss of spinolaminar or facet joint fit.

Classification

This is based on the three principal biomechanical forces resulting in spinal injury:

- axial compression;
- axial distraction;
- translation (due to rotation and shearing) of the forces in a transverse planar direction.

These forces are associated with a number of specific injuries (Table 9.5).

Specific trauma patterns

Compression fractures

These are most frequently characterised by superior end plate depression or anterior wedging. A beak-type projection pointing downwards at the anterior superior edge of the vertebral body (to effectively become a triangular wedge) may be separated and displaced anteriorly. In these cases

Table 9.5 Features of the various spinal injury types.

Description	Characteristics
Wedge compression	Forward flexion causes anterior column failure resulting in fracture, creating vertebral body wedging. Rarely neurological deficit is noted
Stable burst fracture	Consists of anterior and middle column failure under compression without loss of posterior column integrity. Rare
Unstable burst fracture	As above but with disruption of the posterior column resulting in the more common situation of instability with these fractures
Chance fracture	Horizontal vertebral fracture from transverse plane distraction. The fulcrum of the force is anterior to the anterior ligament resulting in the pulling apart of vertebrae by tension
Flexion-distraction	Flexion occurs in the middle column to compress the anterior column until it fails. Middle and posterior columns fail under tension. Tearing of the posterior longitudinal ligament results in potential instability as ligamentum flavum, interspinous and supraspinous ligaments may be damaged
Translation injuries	Disruption and displacement of the spinal column transversely to affect the spinal canal alignment. These may be called dislocations and arise through failure of all three columns following shearing forces

Nine

look for a shearing injury through the laminae and articular facets. Beware of the limbus vertebra that is a normal variant. It is shown as an accessory centre of ossification, outlined by rounded, corticated bone at the antero-superior vertebral margin.

Apophyseal rings are often seen at the antero-superior and inferior vertebral body corners prior to fusion. Prior to ossification, a small indentation of the vertebral body may also be noted in these locations. Neither should be confused with fractures. However, torus-type fractures are seen in childhood at the anterior vertebral body margins.

People with osteoporosis may suffer injury in everyday activities. Acute fracture diagnosis in elderly people is often complicated by superimposed osteoporotic compression injury. This appears to occur earlier in females than males and more frequently in white people than in those of Afro-Caribbean descent. Acute injury is best distinguished by the presence of the following criteria:

- a paraspinous soft tissue mass;
- disruption of bony cortex.

Osteomyelitis of the vertebra is also seen in patients with osteoporosis. This is also seen as a wedge fracture but is accompanied by very severe back pain, pyrexia of unknown origin and raised erythrocyte sedimentation rate. Patients with severe kyphosis often suffer a spontaneous sternal fracture around the manubrio-sternal joint with characteristic

Nine

(a)

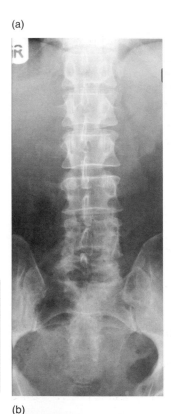

(b)

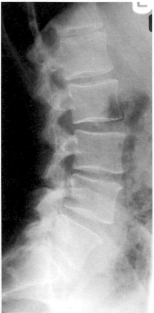

Figure 9.7 Antero-posterior (a) and lateral (b) lumbar spine projections showing burst fracture of L4.

posterior displacement of the superior fragment of the sternum. Multiple osteoporotic collapses are usually contiguous. When collapses are non-contiguous multiple myelomatosis or metastatic/pathological fractures must be excluded. Even where there is a lack of contiguity multiple myeloma should be excluded.

Flexion-distraction

This injury arises, when considered in the three-column model, following excess compression.

- The middle column acts as fulcrum.
- Flexion causes anterior column and structures to undergo compression, generating a wedge deformity.
- The posterior column and structures are subjected to tension causing horizontal fractures and ligament disruption.

Burst fracture (Figures 9.7 and 9.8)

This type of fracture is generated by excess compression axially, to cause splitting off of a postero-superior vertebral body fragment which is pushed into the spinal canal.

- A wedge deformity, often severe, is frequently but not always seen.
- The thoracolumbar junction is the most common site.
- A sagittal fracture of the lower half of the vertebral body is seen in 90% of cases with the involvement of posterior elements in 85%.
- Translational injury components (rotation and shearing to cause ligamentous damage) may be seen in 20% of burst fractures.

Features of burst fracture instability (Figure 9.9) seen radiographically include:

- translational injury components;
- interpediculate distance is increased;

Self-test answer

There appears to be crowding of the spinous processes at the level of L4 and a dense band is evident across the middle of the vertebral body. On the lateral projection a fragment of bone at the postero-inferior corner of the L4 vertebral body is seen to intrude upon the spinal canal. The appearances are consistent with a burst fracture of the fourth lumbar vertebra.

(a)

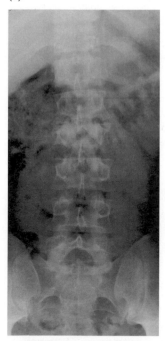

(b)

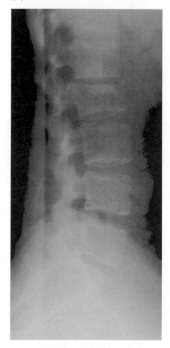

Figure 9.8 Antero-posterior (a) and lateral (b) lumbar spine projections showing burst fracture of L2.

- posterior elements are fractured;
- more than 50% of the vertebral body is subjected to compressive injury.

Review with other modalities such as CT and MRI is advised due to the complex nature of these injuries[4,5].

Fracture-dislocation (translation) injuries

These injuries are generated from a combination of flexion, axial compression and rotational shearing forces. Characteristic features include:

- varying degrees of anterior wedging of the inferior neighbouring vertebral body;
- a triangular fracture fragment sheared from the antero-superior margin of the vertebral body;
- lateral displacement (translation) of the two halves of the fracture components;
- posterior displacement is rare;
- supraspinous and interspinous ligament disruption causing facet joint disruption with laminae and superior facet fractures;
- perching or locking of facets. Here the inferior process of the superior vertebra rides up the superior vertebral processes of the vertebra below and perches close to the end of the lower vertebra's superior intervertebral process;
- superimposition of shearing or rotational forces onto axial compression causing flexion-distraction or pure distraction-type injuries resulting in fractures and dislocation commensurate with these forces.

Translation injuries are very unstable due to the involvement of all three columns. Motor and sensory neurological deficits accompany fracture dislocation injury between the first and eighth thoracic vertebrae. Most common sites of injury of this type are T3–T4 and T5–T6 with T12–L1 (Figure 9.10).

Self-test answer

There is an apparent loss of vertebral body height on the right lateral border of L2 with an associated loss of alignment of the spinous process of L1 and L2. The lateral projection shows a loss of height in the superior vertebral end plate with an associated stepping of the posterior margin of the vertebral body of L2 and resultant bony protrusion into the vertebral canal. Appearances are typical of a burst fracture of the second lumbar vertebra.

Nine

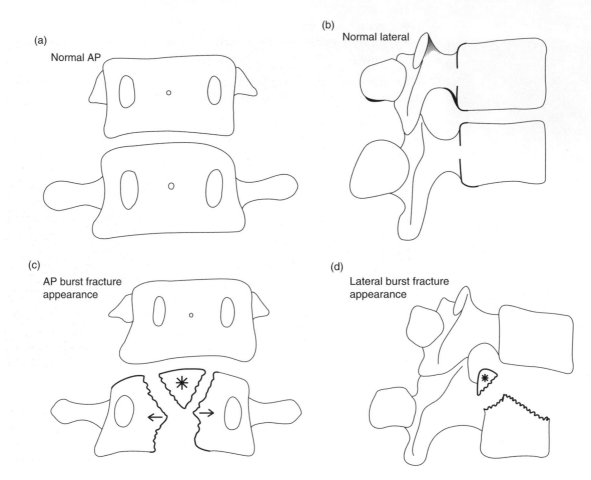

Figure 9.9   The burst fracture of the thoracolumbar spine.

Distraction injuries (Chance fracture)

This unusual fracture demonstrates the following features:

- horizontal splitting of the spinous process and neural arch;
- the splitting ends in an upward curve reaching the upper body surface just anterior to the neural foramen;
- there is usually very little wedging of the vertebral body.

This injury is common among the wearers of lap-type car seat belts (Figure 9.11). The seat belt forms the fulcrum over which the vertebral body splits. A move towards three-point belting systems in vehicles has now helped reduce this phenomenon. The AP view provides two clues in these injuries:

- there is a break of the continuity of usually oval pedicles or tear-shaped spinous process cortices;

(a)   (b)

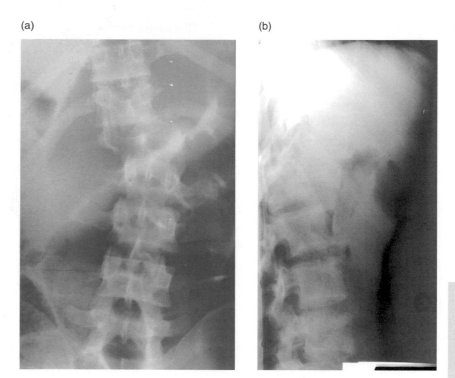

Figure 9.10 Antero-posterior (a) and lateral (b) lumbar spine radiographs showing fracture-dislocation of T12 on L1 (with thanks to the University of Bradford).

Nine

- transverse fracture of the posterior elements or ligament disruption will cause angulation of the superior fracture fragment (or vertebral body) so the posterior elements are no longer superimposed on the body evidenced by 'effective' spinous process fanning.

The lateral view is the confirmatory projection showing the obvious fracture line in the vertebral body, pedicles and spinous process. Ligamentous damage is shown as anterior angulation of the superior vertebral body fragment with posterior element separation.

Due to the method of injury, the term 'seat belt syndrome' has been coined. Collision of the vehicle is head-on at greater than 50 mph to

Self-test answer

There is gross malalignment of the thoracolumbar junction with obvious shifting of thoracic vertebral segment to the right of lumbar vertebra 1. There appears to be a fracture through L1 causing separation of the right superior articular process with resulting anterior displacement of the thoracic segment relative to the lumbar spine. Appearances simulate a translation a Chance-type injury to the spine at T12/L1.

Nine

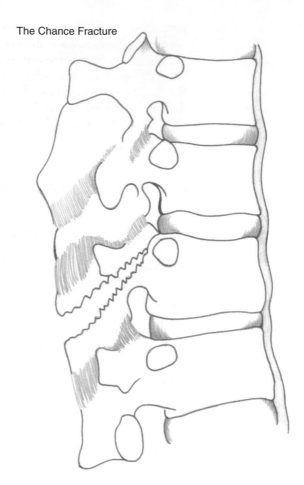

The Chance Fracture

Figure 9.11   The Chance fracture. This fracture literally displays a tearing apart of the bony structures of the posterior vertebral column. It is most commonly noted in lap belt-type injuries.

cause massive deceleration resulting in major force generation around the fulcrum of the lap seat belt. Victims of these accidents generally wear the seat belt around the waist, thus directing force through the lower lumbar spine and into the abdominal viscera. Common associated injuries include:

- transverse abrasions of the lower anterior abdominal wall;
- rupture of the anterior abdominal wall muscles;
- longitudinal laceration of the small bowel;
- rupture/laceration of the spleen, stomach, pancreas in its second and third parts;
- abdominal aorta may be contused;
- injury of the spinal cord and cauda equina;
- transverse spinal fractures;
- rupture of the gravid uterus.

In the UK, because lap belts tend to be fitted as the third seat belt in vehicles, injuries of this nature occur in children[6,7]. As severe trauma is associated with thoracolumbar fractures, failure to diagnose this trauma pattern in the unconscious patient is possible as they are unable to indicate neurological deficit during clinical examination[8].

Finally, the transverse processes of the lumbar spine are a useful indicator of injury as generating a fracture through these bony extensions of the vertebra requires significant force. Although only a minority will display other fractures in the lumbar vertebra, scrutinise the film for signs that other damage may be present that would be fully revealed in a CT[9].

Injuries of the cervical spine

Radiographic evidence of injury

Soft tissues

Haemorrhage or oedema will cause an increase in the dimensions of the retropharyngeal soft tissue. As these reactions follow injury, underlying fracture or dislocation of the cervical spine could be inferred as seen in Table 9.6. Table 9.7 gives the suggested upper limits of the soft tissue dimensions anterior to C3 and C4. **However,** retropharyngeal soft tissue dimensions are not reliable indicators because of the great overlap between normal and abnormal. Many patients with fractures do not display an increase in retropharyngeal soft tissue width[10].

Malalignment

Four convex lines of the cervical spine (Figure 9.12) are useful indicators of correct position from the lateral view:

Table 9.6 Retropharyngeal soft tissue dimensions at various cervical levels.

Position/level	Dimension
Anterior to arch of C1	10 mm
Anterior to base of C2	5 mm
Anterior to C3 and upper margin of C4	7 mm
Anterior to C6 and C7	20 mm

Table 9.7 Soft tissue dimensions anterior to C3/C4 related to probability of injury.

Dimension	Likelihood of injury
Up to 5 mm	Injury unlikely
5 mm to 7 mm	Injury possible but rare
7 mm to 10 mm	Injury is likely
Over 10 mm	Injury is probable

Nine

Nine

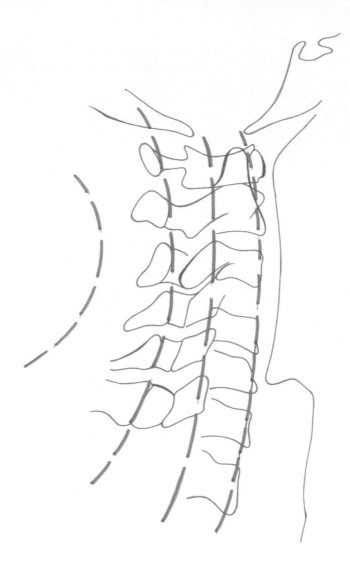

Figure 9.12 The cervical spine curves. Note how the lines follow the smooth curves of the vertebral column on the lateral projection. The spinous process curve has been deliberately separated from the tips of the processes to reinforce the idea that normal variation may lead to mis-representation of what is seen in the image.

- anterior border of vertebral bodies – useful until degenerative changes cause osteophytic spur formation;
- posterior vertebral body cortices;
- anterior margin of the junction of spinous processes/laminae;
- the spinous process tips display wide normal variation among individuals so exercise caution when using this indicator.

Similar imaginary lines may be used on the AP film. They should be straight or gently curved and aid review where spasm causes difficulty in assessment on the lateral projection. These are along the lateral vertebral margins and the spinous processes in the midline.

Abrupt disruption/angulation of these lines will alert the viewer to a problem. Lateral mass fractures or facet joint dislocations will cause

(a)

(b)

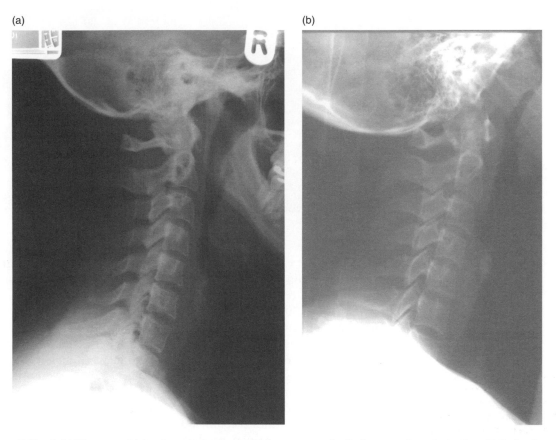

Figure 9.13 (a,b) The normal lateral cervical spine projection compared with the normal cervical spine displaying loss of lordosis.

disruption of the gently undulating line that highlights the alignment of the masses. Remember, however, normal spinal lordosis (Figure 9.13) can be lost or slightly reversed in patients with muscle spasm of the neck.

In the open-mouth projection (Figure 9.14) particular care should be exercised to ensure the lateral masses of C1 are equidistant from the odontoid peg. Any discrepancy should initiate a search for overhanging of C1 lateral masses beyond the lateral margins of C2. Suspect a cervical ring fracture if this is the case otherwise the appearance may be ascribed to rotation of the image or normal variance in the subject. Flexion occurs around C5/C6 in adults and at C2/C3 in children. In

Self-test answer

Trace out the lines and relationships of the normal cervical spine relative to the example of the loss of lordosis.

Nine

(a)   (b)

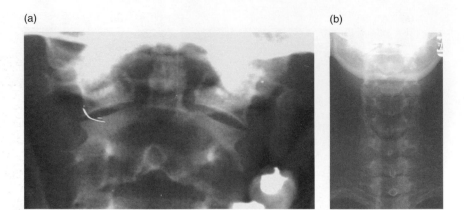

Figure 9.14   (a) The normal open-mouth (OM) projection. (b) The normal AP cervical spine projection.

children a normal variant that may be seen is a small physiological anterior offset of C2 on C3 and sometimes of C3 on C4. A mis-diagnosis of subluxation, due to misinterpretation of this phenomenon, may be made in patients up to 30 years of age.

The interspinous ligament (and therefore posterior column injury) is revealed as increased interspinous distance due to spinous process fanning on the lateral view. Rotational malalignment is suggested by the displacement of the spinous process to the affected side on the AP film. Although plain film imaging is the method widely employed as a first-line approach to detect the signs discussed above and the patterns below[11], some authorities recommend a wider use of CT to fully elucidate injuries that may or may not be visible on an initial examination[12].

The upper cervical spine

Atlas (C1) – neural arch fracture

Bilateral vertical fracture (Figure 9.15) through the neural arch is the most common fracture of C1. Hyperextension of the head compresses the C1 neural arch between the occiput and the neural arch of C2. The open-mouth view will show if the lateral masses have spread out, as is evident in Jefferson's fracture. Horizontal fracture of the anterior arch of atlas may occur – it is usually accompanied by an odontoid peg

Self-test answer

Check the alignment of the lateral masses of C1 relative to C2. This image in particular raises the issues associated with rotation in the open-mouth projection.

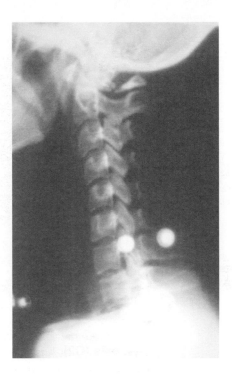

Figure 9.15 Bilateral neural arch fracture of C1.

Nine

fracture. Lateral plain films/tomography show this best. CT may miss the lesion as the scan may lie in the plane of the fracture.

Jefferson's fracture

These are burst fractures of the ring of C1 and are defined as comminuted fractures of the ring involving both anterior and posterior arches. Transmission of force from the skull downwards causes fracture and disruption of the weak anterior and posterior C1 arches to spread apart the lateral masses[13]. Confirmation on the AP projection is assured where the lateral masses of C1 overhang the lateral portion of C2. This is helpful in those films produced with apparent unilateral C1/C2 joint space widening which may be a normal variant or purely a rotated image. Figure 9.16 shows the open-mouth cervical spine projection revealing a burst fracture of C1.

Self-test answer

There is a break in the ring of C1. There is a loss of the normal cervical lordosis and evidence of the presence of a neck collar as revealed by the white artefacts at the level of C7 and at the extreme anterior of the radiograph at the level of T1.

Nine

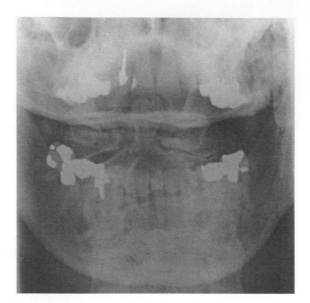

Figure 9.16 The open-mouth cervical spine projection revealing a burst fracture of C1.

The axis (C2)

Approximately 15% of cervical fractures involve the axis. Of these, 40% are seen with head injuries and 18% with other cervical spine injuries. Twenty-five per cent of C2 fractures are hangman's fractures and 55% are odontoid fractures. The remainder are fractures of the body, lateral mass, spinous process or single fractures of the neural arch.

Hangman's fracture (Figure 9.17)
Named after the injury caused to the cervical spine by judicial hanging, it occurs following hyperextension of the head on the neck but may occur following hyperflexion and compression. Defined as a traumatic spondylolisthesis of the axis, fractures of the neural arch of axis or fractures of the ring of the axis are seen. Injury occurs when transmission of the force of hyperextension of the head through the C2 pedicles onto the apophyseal joints causes a fracture anterior to the inferior facet of C2. Tension may also disrupt the anterior longitudinal ligament. Lateral films show the injury best (Figure 9.18).

Self-test answer

Although the projection is sub-optimal, it can be seen that the lateral masses of C1 overhang the lateral borders of the body of C2 on the right. This is indicative of a burst or Jefferson's fracture of C1.

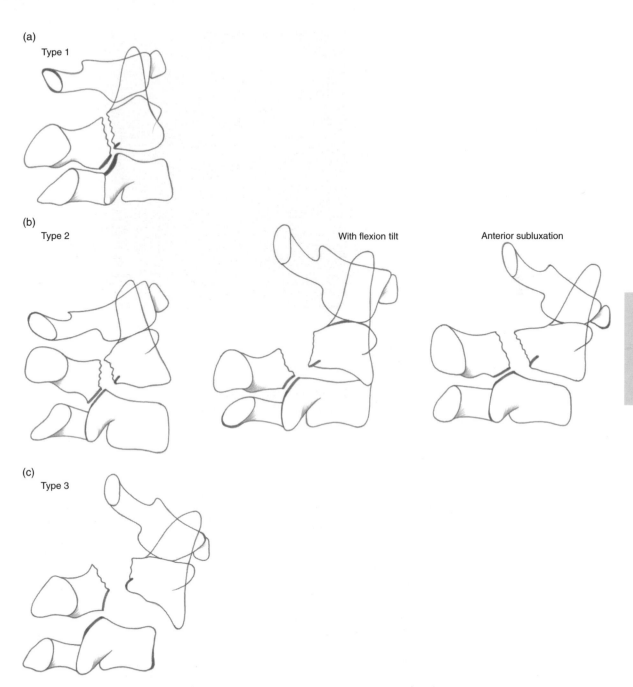

Figure 9.17 (a–c) Hangman's fractures according to Effendi.

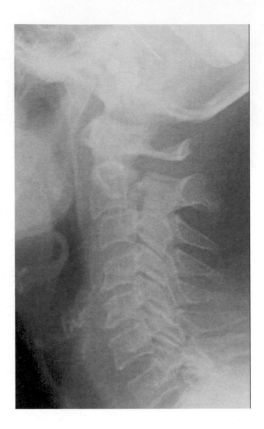

Figure 9.18   Lateral cervical spine radiograph: hangman's fracture.

Odontoid peg fractures (Figures 9.19 and 9.20)

Odontoid peg fractures usually occur through the base of the peg. If it has an oblique extension into the vertebral body anteriorly, it may not be seen on the open-mouth view. Anderson and D'Alonzo have proposed a classification of odontoid peg fractures consisting of three types (see also Figure 9.21).

- Type 1 – an oblique fracture linked to the peg; 4% of these injuries.

Self-test answer

There is an obvious bilateral break of the pars interarticularis of C2. A loss of the normal cervical lordosis is noted with apparent forward slip of C2 on C3. There also appears to be a widening of the intervertebral relation between C3 and C4 which would be possible in this type of injury. Appearances are indicative of a hangman's-type fracture of C2.

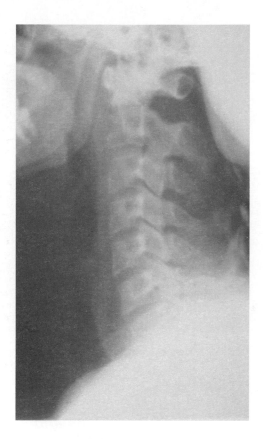

Figure 9.19 Lateral cervical spine projection showing fracture of the base of the odontoid peg with some loss of alignment.

- Type 2 – a transverse fracture at the base of the peg accounts for 66% of odontoid peg injuries.
- Type 3 – an oblique fracture at the base of the peg extending into the body; 30% of these injuries.

The os odontoideum is a normal variant that may be confused with a minimal type 1 fracture. Projection of the upper incisors may also confuse the appearance by creating an impression of a vertical split in the upper portion of the dens.

Self-test answer

There is a lucency extending across the base of the odontoid peg and associated loss of continuity of the cortices of the dens at this level. There is a suggestion that some forward slippage of the odontoid peg has also occurred. All signs point towards a type 2 fracture of the dens.

Nine

(a)   (b)

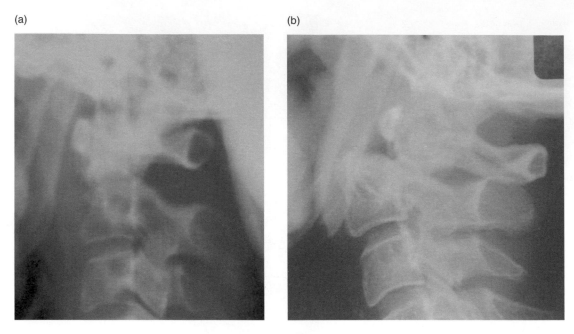

Figure 9.20 (a,b) Further images of odontoid peg fractures showing the variation in presentation that may be encountered.

Dislocations and subluxations

Atlanto-occipital dislocations (Figure 9.22)

These injuries are usually fatal due to disruption of the medulla oblongata. Survivors have been reported, three times more frequently in children than adults. Lateral films show the anatomical relationships that best inform the viewer of potential problems. A prominent soft tissue swelling usually accompanies the injury. The injury has three forms:

- dislocation of the head anterior to the cervical spine;
- less commonly there is a separation of the occiput from the atlas by distraction;
- rarely the head dislocates posteriorly relative to the spine.

Atlanto-axial dislocation (Figure 9.23)

The most commonly dislocated area of the cranio-vertebral junction, this injury is associated with:

- rheumatoid-type arthritides;
- Down's syndrome; and
- may occur transiently following severe head and neck infections that result in ligamentous laxity.

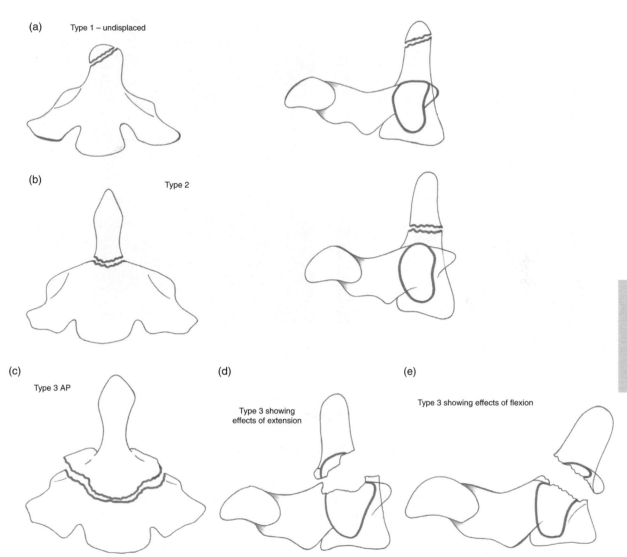

(a) Type 1 – undisplaced

(b) Type 2

(c) Type 3 AP

(d) Type 3 showing effects of extension

(e) Type 3 showing effects of flexion

Figure 9.21 (a–e) Classification of odontoid peg fractures.

The injury is revealed by an increase in the distance between the posterior cortex of the anterior arch of the atlas and the anterior cortex of the odontoid peg. This is known as the pre-dental space, and normal dimensions are:

- adults – 2.5 mm;
- children – 5.0 mm.

Dislocation may occur in trauma though this is rare and arises from hyperflexion and shearing forces disrupting the transverse ligament of the atlas. Usually considered a component of Jefferson's fracture, any

Nine

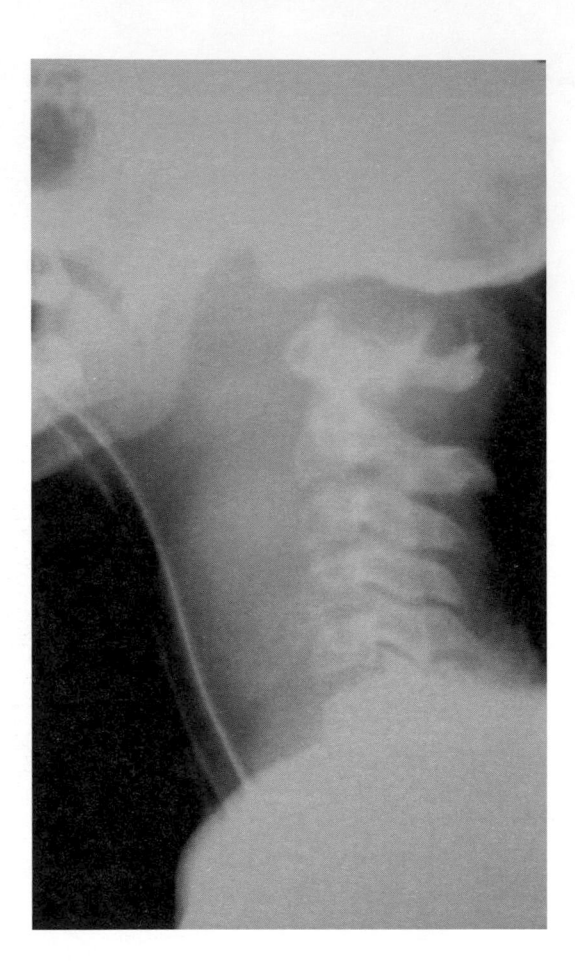

Figure 9.22 Lateral cervical spine displaying atlanto-occipital dislocation.

evidence of dislocation should be accompanied by a search for associated fracture(s). Lateral films in flexion are the best indicators of the problem. However, as stated earlier, the availability of other imaging modalities, in the presence of clinical neurological change, suggests that this approach is a controversial form of imaging.

Self-test answer

There is an obvious separation of the atlas from the occipital condyles of the skull with associated massive swelling of the soft tissues anterior to the cervical spine. These appearances are consistent with atlanto-occipital dislocation. The airway is protected by what appears to be an endotracheal tube. Artefacts from a neck collar are seen at C4/5, C2/3 and anterior to the odontoid peg. Being a sub-optimal projection it is difficult to say whether further injury exists below the level of C6.

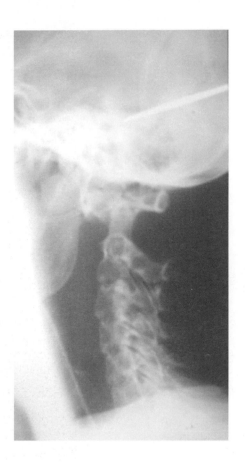

Figure 9.23 Lateral cervical spine projection displaying atlanto-axial dislocation.

Nine

Neurological injury

Why are there relatively few neurological injuries related to the cranio-vertebral junction? This is because the spinal cord occupies about 50% of the canal space and so is afforded some protection. Also, in Jefferson's, hangman's and ring of atlas fractures, due to the mechanics

Self-test answer

There is an obvious widening of the joint between C1 and C2 with a relative anterior shift of C1 to the rest of the spinal column. There is some swelling of the soft tissue anterior to the cervical spine with evidence of airway protection by an endotracheal tube. The remaining cervical vertebrae have an unusual appearance and there appears to be a ventriculo-peritoneal shunt *in situ.* Is there history of any other associated syndrome in this patient?

Table 9.8   Characteristics of cervical spine flexion injuries.

Type of injury	Characteristics
Anterior wedge	Relatively minor loss of height at anterior section of vertebral body
Hyperflexion strain	Posterior ligaments are damaged when there is anterior subluxation of the vertebral body. There may be increased intervertebral disc height with spinous process fanning and local kyphosis
Pillar fracture	Hyperflexion and rotation or distraction cause force focusing mainly on the side of rotation to fracture through the articular pillar[14]
Unilateral locked facet	Flexion, distraction and rotation cause the facets to ride up to create an appearance of facet overlap on the lateral image. May be called a 'bow-tie' sign
Bilateral locked facets	Significant flexion and distraction to cause the related facets to ride over each other so that they become disarticulated. The vertebral body of the upper vertebra is displaced approximately 50% anteriorly relative to the lower vertebra on the lateral image
Clay shoveller	Avulsion of spinous process of C6 or C7 following excessive muscular load during a flexing movement
Tear-drop burst fracture	Comminuted vertebral body fracture with a large antero-inferior triangular fragment. The posterior part of the vertebral body may be displaced into the spinal canal, resulting in neural damage. Most severe form of flexion injury to the cervical spine

of bone movement – centrifugal displacement in Jefferson's fractures and posterior displacement in C1 posterior arch and C2 neural arch fractures – the spinal canal is increased in size, thus protecting the cord and avoiding neurological damage.

The lower cervical spine

Flexion injuries

The range of flexion injuries (Figures 9.24–9.27) is reviewed in Table 9.8. Where severe flexion is experienced the cervical vertebrae may ride over each other to generate a bilateral facet dislocation (Figures 9.28 and 9.29). If less force is experienced perched facets may occur. However, there is an overlap of adjacent vertebral bodies in the region of 50% in both types of injury. Where a rotatory component is also experienced during flexion unilateral dislocation of the facet joint may occur and generate the bow-tie sign. In the frontal projection the spinous process moves toward the side that has been dislocated as the vertebra twists out of position (Figure 9.30).

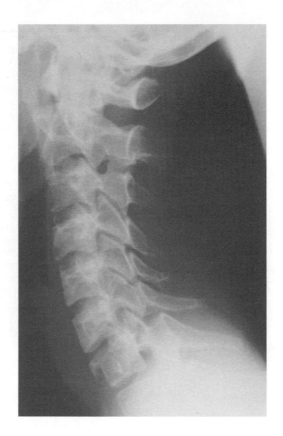

Figure 9.24 Lateral cervical spine projection that reveals a flexion wedge fracture of C7.

Nine

Extension injuries

The signs may be quite subtle and include:

- pre-vertebral soft tissue swelling;
- widened intervertebral disc space at the anterior portion of the bodies;
- posterior body displacement;
- vacuum phenomenon at the annulus fibrosus in the absence of degenerative disease. This is a gas stripe in the intervertebral disc space that comes about when nitrogen in solution in the body becomes gaseous following a pressure change in the disc due to a

Self-test answer

There is a loss of the anterior vertebral body height of C7 and an apparent forward movement of C6 on C7. There is the suggestion that a lucent line extends into the vertebral body from the anterior edge of the wedging of C7. The appearances are indicative of a flexion wedge fracture of C7.

Nine

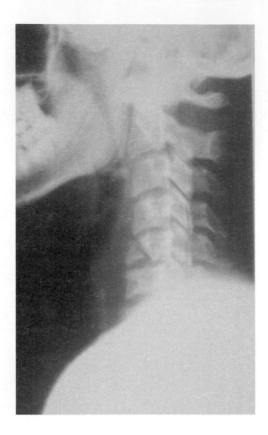

Figure 9.25   Lateral cervical spine projection showing a hyperflexion tear-drop injury to C5.

change in its volume. The disc volume change occurs following overextension.

As with other pathological processes, ankylosing spondylitis severely weakens bone. When coupled with the tendency of the disease to render the spinal column into, effectively, a tube, it can be seen that patients with this disease will be prone to more serious injuries in simple flexion/extension (whiplash) mechanisms. Careful scrutiny is required using the above search approaches; however, the observer must take account of changes in bone construction as subtle injuries are difficult to detect[15].

Self-test answer

There is a loss of the normal lordosis of the cervical spine. The C5 vertebral body has an oblique lucency passing through it from the antero-superior corner of the vertebral body to the midpoint of the inferior end plate. The appearances are indicative of a hyperflexion tear-drop injury of the C5 vertebra. Assessment for vertebral stability is advised.

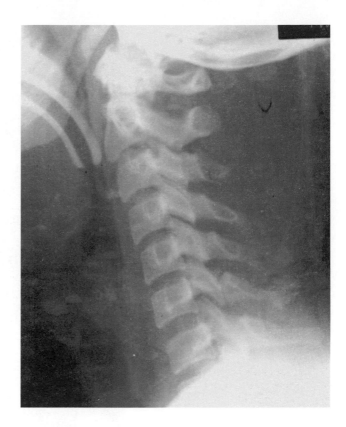

Figure 9.26 Lateral cervical spine projection showing fracture with subluxation at C6/7.

The clay shoveller's fracture (Figure 9.31)

An injury purely in the spinous process, this comes about from the tension created by muscular pull on the spinous processes and takes its name from the cause of injury – heavy digging work over a long period.

Self-test answer

The patient's airway is protected by an endotracheal device resting at the level of C2/3. There is a loss of the normal cervical lordosis. Closer examination reveals an apparent widening of the intervertebral disc space at the level of C6/7. There are also lucencies in the posterior vertebral structures of C6 that seem to extend across the pedicle and anterior to the spinolaminar line, indicating a double fracture across the vertebral pillar. All these signs should be treated with suspicion of fracture with residual subluxation from an earlier dislocation. Further imaging with CT is advised.

Nine

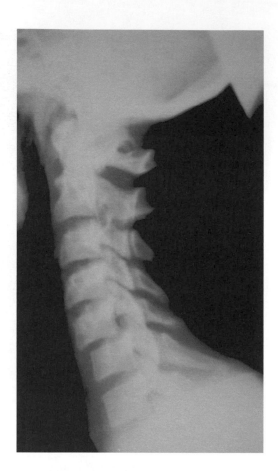

Figure 9.27 Lateral cervical spine projection revealing resultant subluxation with an associated fracture of the C5 pedicle.

Imagine that the heavy clay prevents a person from lifting the shovel without excessive muscular force. The obvious sequela of this is the fracture of the muscular insertion, that is, the pathognomic break of the spinous process[16].

Self-test answer

There is an apparent loss of intervertebral disc height at the C5/6 joint space with an associated forward slippage of C5 on C6 of approximately one quarter of the C5 vertebral body length. There is also an apparent lucency at the junction of the pedicle with the posterior vertebral body surface that is highly suggestive of the presence of a fracture. Further confirmatory imaging is advised.

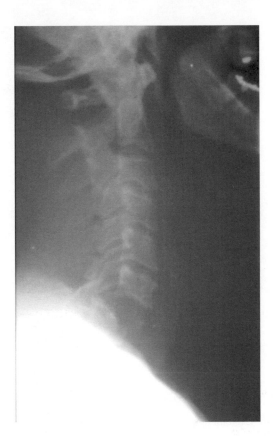

Figure 9.28 Lateral cervical spine projection showing bilateral facet dislocation of C6 on C7 and associated fracture of C7.

Radiographic signs of instability

Where instability is suspected following an injury, the following indicators are useful in the evaluation of the cervical spine:

- widening of intervertebral disc space in all stress views;
- fanning of the spinous process;

Self-test answer

There is a widening and gross malalignment of the C6/7 intervertebral joint. There is also a large wedge fracture of the superior vertebral border of C7. The inferior intervertebral processes of C6 now lie anterior to the superior intervertebral articular processes. These appearances would indicate that the patient has undergone a severe hyperflexion injury resulting in a teardrop-type wedge fracture of C7 and an associated bilateral facet dislocation of C6 on C7. Further imaging is advised.

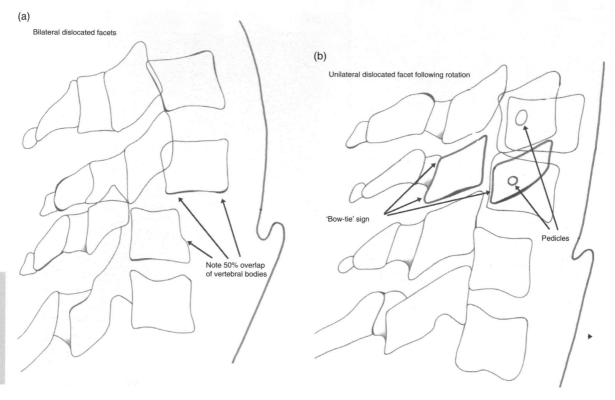

Figure 9.29   (a,b) Bilateral and unilateral facet dislocation features.

- disruption of facets;
- horizontal displacement of one body on another more than 3.5 mm;
- severe injury, e.g. multiple fractures at one segment.

Some considerations in children

As indicated for adults violent force is often involved in causing injury. Care should be exercised in ruling out secondary ossification centres as a cause for concern. However, the synchondrosis (cartilaginous plate) of C2 may be sheared during rapid deceleration accidents such as in appropriately restrained back seat car passengers in a head-on collision[17]. Rarely does child abuse generate enough force to cause injuries such as fracture dislocations of the lower cervical spine or hangman's-type injuries although it is wise to keep this pattern in mind when reviewing cases of suspected non-accidental injury[18,19]. More likely is the failure to make an association between the very young child and falls from heights less than 2 m which cause upper cervical injuries that may not produce significant clinical signs[20].

(a) (b)

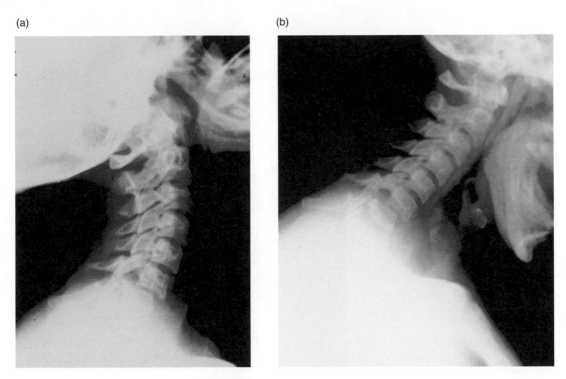

Figure 9.30 (a,b) Flexion and extension lateral projections showing the resultant instability and extent of subluxation.

Image artefacts and normal variants (Figures 9.32 and 9.33)

Common image artefacts frequently result in the production of a sub-optimal image, making assessment difficult. The basic need to image the traumatised cervical spine in the horizontal beam position, often with associated vascular lines and airway support tubes in situ, results in the production of the sub-optimal image. When reviewing the film take care to account for these appearances, many of which are seen in the associated images.

Self-test answer

Comparison of the extension and flexion projections (9.30 a and b, respectively) shows an apparent increase in the size of the joint space widening and further anterior movement of C6 on C7 in the flexion projection. This is suggestive of severe disruption of the posterior ligamentous structures.
NB: Had there been the suggestion that this was likely via clinical assessment or earlier imaging, performance of this type of examination would be ill advised.

Nine

Nine

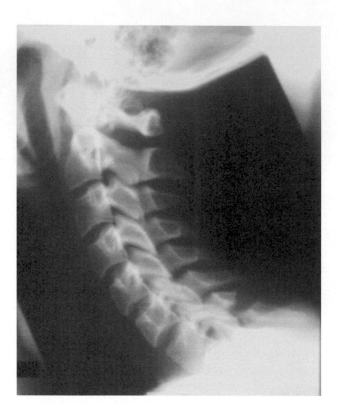

Figure 9.31 Lateral cervical spine projection showing clay shoveller-type injury of the spinous process.

The horizontal beam projection may generate an image of a spine that has lost its apparently normal cervical lordosis – often taken as an indicator of underlying traumatic changes. Remember to look for other indicators that will confirm definite injury. The mach line (which comes about due to rapid change in subject contrast of the body of the patient being examined relative to kV/mAS factors used in the imaging process) across the open-mouth projection could be confused as a base of odontoid peg fracture. Scrutinise carefully to see if this dark line extends beyond the cortical margins of the odontoid peg, as this would confirm this image artefact is present. A similar feature may be noted where a gap between the incisors is projected over the peg to give the appearance

Self-test answer

An obvious fracture extends across the origin of the spinous process of C7. Its extension would appear to communicate with the lamina of the vertebra; however, there does not appear to be any loss of cervical lordosis or alignment of the associated vertebrae. The appearance is consistent with a 'clay shovelling' mechanism of injury although a direct blow may produce a similar appearance.

(a)

(b)

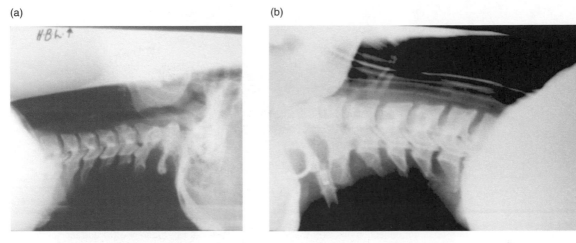

Figure 9.32 (a,b) Lateral cervical spine radiographs showing positional variation and artefacts.

of a fracture. Again it should be possible to exclude this as a fracture due to extension of the line beyond the apex of the axis.

The bifid spinous process has been cited as a cause for concern on the lower cervical spine images, giving an impression that the vertebra has rotated out of position following unilateral dislocation – look carefully to assure yourself that this is a normal variant. In a similar way the pre-dental space has been identified as a cause for careful scrutiny along with physiological offsetting of C3 and C4 at various ages.

Finally, the os odontoideum should be remembered as a cause for concern in the dens. Usually forming a minor portion of the upper part of the peg, this secondary ossification centre will be apparent through careful examination of the bone edges. Secondary ossification points

Self-test answer (a)

Note loss of normal cervical lordosis due to projection. Remember, however, that muscle spasm or the patient guarding the injured neck may generate appearances like this that should not be dismissed out of hand as they may represent an actual injury.

Self-test answer (b)

Take note of the positions of various lines introduced in the resuscitation room. They can overlie and mask soft tissue interfaces that may be of diagnostic value.

Nine

(a)   (b)   (c)

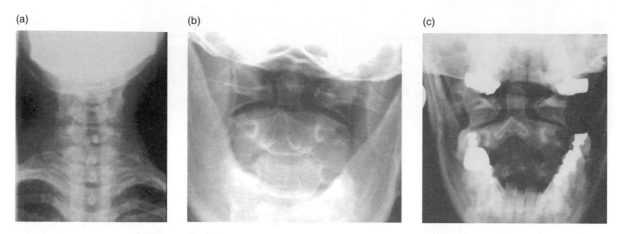

Figure 9.33   (a–c) The antero-posterior projection showing the bifid spinous process (a), mach line (b) and incisor line (c).

tend to be rounded off rather than forming, typically, a jigsaw fit where fracture fragments are in close apposition.

References

1   Hu, R., Mustard, C.A. and Burns, C. (1996) Epidemiology of incident spinal fracture in a complete population. *Spine* **21**(4), 492–9.
2   Wnaisch, R.D. (1996) Vertebral fracture epidemiology. *Bone* **18**(3 Suppl), 179S–183S.
3   Biyani, A., Ebraheim, N.A. and Lu, J. (1996) Thoracic spine fractures in patients older than 50 years. *Clinical Orthopaedics and Related Research* **328**, 190–3.
4   Saifuddin, A., Noordeen, H., Taylor, B.A., *et al.* (1996) The role of imaging in the diagnosis and management of thoracolumbar burst frac-

Self-test answer

Note how the bifid spinous process can be misconstrued as either a fracture or the rotated component of a single facet dislocation.

Self-test answer

Note how the mach (b) and incisor (c) line can be projected over the odontoid peg to generate an impression of fracture presence.

tures: current concepts and review of the literature. *Skeletal Radiology* **25**(7), 603–13.

5 Petersilge, C.A. and Emery, S.E. (1996) Thoracolumbar burst fracture evaluating stability. *Seminars in Ultrasound, CT & MR* **17**(2), 105–13.

6 Voss, L., Cole, P.A. and D'Amato, C. (1996) Paediatric chance fractures from lap belts: unique case report of three in one accident. *Journal of Orthopaedic Trauma* **10**(6), 421–8.

7 Statter, M.B. and Vargish, T. (1998) The spectrum of lap belt injuries sustained by two cousins in the same motor vehicle crash. *Journal of Trauma* **45**(4), 835–7.

8 Stanislas, M.J., Latham, J.M., Porter, K.M., *et al.* (1998) A high risk group for thoracolumbar fractures. *Injury* **29**(1), 15–18.

9 Krueger, M.A., Green, D.A., Hoyt, D., *et al.* (1996) Overlooked spine injuries associated with lumbar transverse process fractures. *Clinical Orthopaedics and Related Research* **327**, 191–5.

10 Herr, C.H., Ball, P.A., Sargent, S.K., *et al.* (1998) Sensitivity of prevertebral soft tissue measurement of C3 for detection of cervical spine fractures and dislocations. *American Journal of Emergency Medicine* **16**(4), 346–9.

11 Tehranzadeh, J. and Palmer, S. (1996) Imaging of cervical spine trauma. *Seminars in Ultrasound, CT & MR* **17**(2), 93–104.

12 Nunez, D.B., Zuluaga, A., Fuentes-Bernado, D.A., *et al.* (1996) Cervical spine trauma: how much more do we learn by routinely using helical CT? *Radiographics* **16**(6), 1307–18.

13 Beckner, M.A., Heggeness, M.H. and Doherty, B.J. (1998) A biomechanical study of Jefferson's fractures. *Spine* **23**(17), 1832–6.

14 Shanmuganathan, K., Mirvis, S.E., Dowe, M., *et al.* (1996) Traumatic isolation of the cervical articular pillar: imaging observations in 21 patients. *American Journal of Roentgenology* **166**(4), 897–902.

15 Olerud, C., Frost, A. and Bring, J. (1996) Spinal fractures in patients with ankylosing spondylitis. *European Spine Journal* **5**(1), 51–5.

16 Dellestable, F. and Gaucher, A. (1998) Clay-shoveler's fracture. Stress fracture of the lower cervical and upper thoracic spinous processes. *Revue du Rhumatisme (English edition)* **65**(10), 575–82.

17 Blauth, M., Scmidt, U., Otte, D., *et al.* (1996) Fractures of the odontoid process in small children: biomechanical analysis and report of three cases. *European Spine Journal* **5**(1), 63–70.

18 Rooks, V.J., Sisler, C. and Burton, B. (1998) Cervical injury in child abuse: a report of two cases. *Pediatric Radiology* **28**(3), 193–5.

19 Kleinman, P.K. and Shelton, Y.A. (1997) Hangman's fracture in an abused infant: imaging features. *Pediatric Radiology* **27**(9), 776–7.

20 Schwartz, G.R., Wright, S.W., Fein, J.A., *et al.* (1997) Pediatric cervical spine injury sustained in falls from low heights. *Annals of Emergency Medicine* **30**(3), 249–52.

Nine

10 Pelvic Fractures

Renata Eyres

Introduction

Pelvic fractures are relatively uncommon; however, complications with the contents of the pelvis may arise following severe injury[1,2]. These include damage to the lower urinary tract or complications arising from bleeding from the large vessels.

The inferior or 'true' pelvis is separated from the superior or 'false' pelvis by the iliopectineal line. The superior pelvis is actually part of the abdomen and consists mainly of the iliac wings. The inferior pelvis contains the lower urinary tract, the pelvic peritoneal reflection and pelvic small bowel loops, distal colon, reproductive organs and the pelvic vessels and nerves.

The pelvic ring (Figure 10.1) has no inherent stability and relies on ligamentous support. Stability is provided by:

- the iliolumbar ligaments;
- the dorsal sacroiliac ligaments and anterior sacroiliac;
- the sacrotuberous ligaments;
- the sacrospinous ligaments;
- the postero-superior interosseous ligaments.

Systematic review of the injured pelvis should be undertaken in every case as outlined in Appendix 3.

Classification of pelvic fractures

Pelvic fractures may be classified as either minor/isolated fractures or major/displaced fractures with disruption of the pelvic ring. Their

Figure 10.1 The normal pelvis (pelvic image courtesy of xray2000.co.uk). Ligaments are shown as follows: black lines (anterior sacroiliac ligament), dotted lines (sacrotuberal ligament), dotted arrow (sacrospinal ligament), arrow (posterior sacroiliac ligaments, seen mainly in posterior view). Bony anatomy is as follows: sacrum (A), iliac crest (B), anterior superior iliac spine (C), sacroiliac joint (D), anterior inferior iliac spine (E), acetabular joint space (F), head of femur (G), greater trochanter (H), lesser trochanter (I), intertrochanteric line (J), superior pubic ramus (K), inferior pubic ramus (L), symphysis pubis (M), obturator foramen (N), ischial tuberosity (O), ischial spine (P), iliac wing (Q).

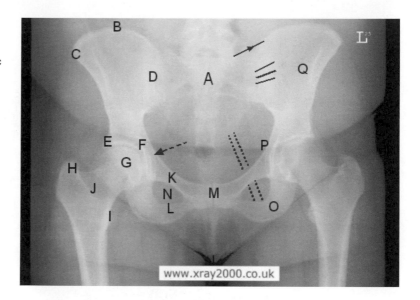

stability can be judged by fracture pattern and knowledge of the mechanism of injury and the anatomy of the pelvic ligaments[3].

Minor (stable) pelvic fractures

These are fractures where the pelvic ring remains stable. Usually there is a fracture of an individual bone without a break in the continuity of the pelvic ring. They include avulsion fractures of:

- anterior superior iliac spine (ASIS);
- the anterior inferior iliac spine (AIIS);
- the ischial tuberosity;
- the ilium.

Avulsion fractures (Figure 10.2) are fairly common sporting injuries in long jumpers, hurdlers and gymnasts[4].

Single breaks in the pelvic ring may occur and present as:

- fracture of two ipsilateral rami;
- subluxation of or fracture near the symphysis pubis;
- subluxation of or fracture near the sacroiliac joint.

Sacral fractures may be isolated, usually transverse and result from a direct blow. When seen as part of more complex trauma, they are normally vertical[5]. They may result from sacral insufficiency due to osteoporosis, when they are again vertical and appear as a dense line that runs parallel to the sacroiliac joint.

When the pelvic ring remains intact following injury there should be no damage to the pelvic contents.

Ten

(a)

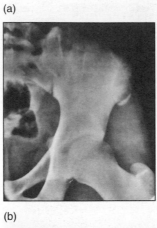

(b)

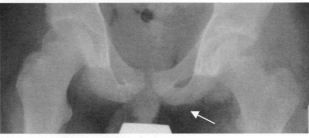

(c)

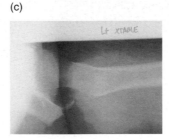

Figure 10.2 (a) Avulsion injury to the anterior superior iliac spine via sartorius. (b, c) Avulsion of the ischial tuberosity.

Major (unstable) pelvic fractures

These are fractures where there is disruption of the pelvic ring in two or more places, resulting in displacement of the pelvis (Figure 10.3). The common causes of major pelvic trauma may be further divided into three main groups, based upon the mechanism of injury[6].

Self-test answer (a)

A flake of bone that appears to originate from the left anterior superior iliac spine region suggests that there has been an avulsion injury, probably caused by the pull of the sartorius muscle.

(a)

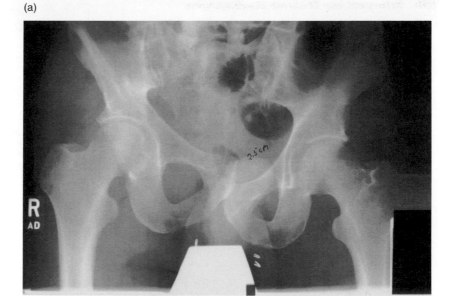

(b)

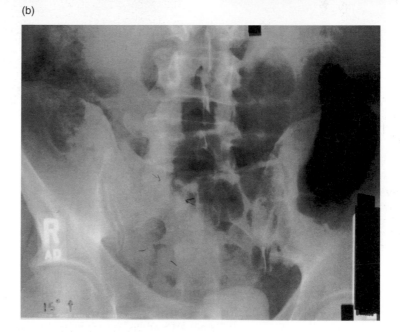

Figure 10.3 (a, b) Multiple pelvic injuries.

Self test answer

Further to the above appearances (a) and allowing for overlying bowel gas shadows, there is apparent widening of the left sacroiliac joint commensurate with disruption of the anterior sacroiliac ligaments.

Self test answer

There is disruption of the symphysis pubis whereby the left side rests inferior to the right with slight over-riding.

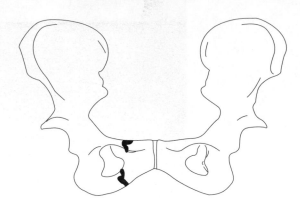

Figure 10.4 Pubic rami fracture.

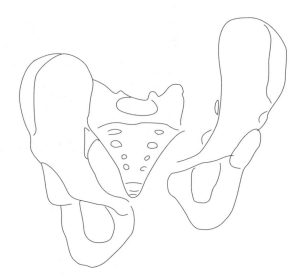

Figure 10.5 Vertical shear fracture.

Ten

Antero-posterior force fractures

These occur where antero-posterior compression is applied to the pelvis, such as when a pedestrian is hit head on by a car or a person is crushed between two objects. Fractures of the pubic rami, diastasis of the symphysis pubis and disruption of the anterior sacroiliac ligaments follow this force vector. All four pubic rami may be fractured (Figure 10.4) and displaced posteriorly, although the pelvic ring may be stable. Such injuries may result in damage to the bladder and urethra (see diastasis fractures, p. 246).

Lateral force fractures

The most common mechanism of injury, resulting in interal rotation of the affected hemipelvis, dislocated or overlapping fractures of pubic rami and/or symphysis pubis, and inpacted lateral wing of sacrum fractures.

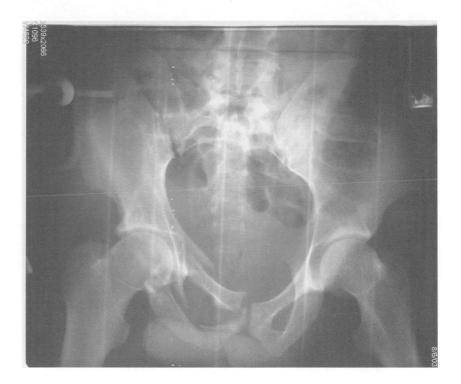

Figure 10.6 Vertical fracture of the right hemipelvis.

Vertical shear fractures

These often result from a fall from a height. The pubic rami may be fractured and the hemipelvis displaced superiorly (Figures 10.5 and 10.6). These are unstable fractures which may cause damage to the pelvic viscera and produce neurovascular complications.

- Malgaigne fracture – consists of fractured sacrum with ipsilateral superior and inferior pubic rami fractures (Figure 10.7).
- Straddle fracture – involves both superior and inferior pubic rami bilaterally (Figure 10.8).

Self test answer

A fracture line is seen to traverse, vertically, the right iliac wing approximately 2 cm lateral to the sacroiliac joint. Further fractures are noted through the superior and inferior pubic rami with an extension through the inferior ischial ramus apparently into the acetabulum. The symphysis pubis appears to have been disrupted. Further imaging, i.e. CT or specialised plain film projections, are required to fully evaluate such fractures.

Ten

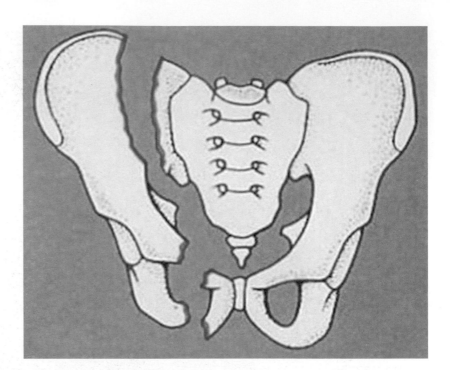

Figure 10.7 Malgaigne fracture.

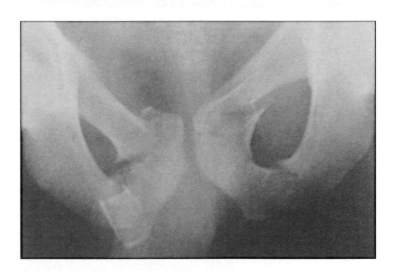

Figure 10.8 Straddle fracture of the pubic complex.

Diastasis or book fractures

These are where the pelvis is 'opened out' (Figure 10.9). The diastasis is usually at the symphysis pubis, but may also be associated with diastasis of the sacroiliac joint and massive retro-pelvic haemorrhage. In severe injuries all the above may occur, particularly following a high-velocity impact. The radiographic appearance may be asymmetry of the iliac wings, one appearing broader and flatter than the other. Computed

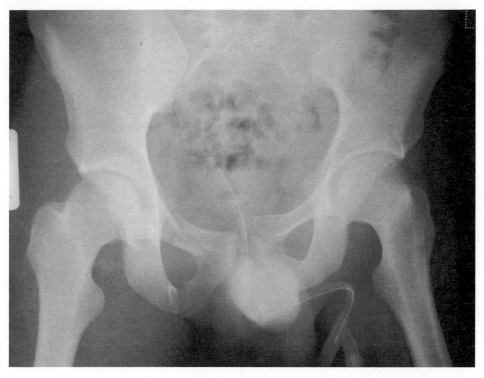

Figure 10.9   A fracture of superior and inferior pubic rami on the right side is combined with diastasis of the sacroiliac joint on the left, and separation of the symphysis pubis. Note the presence of a urinary catheter. An open book fracture also has a characteristic widening of the symphysis, which can often be extreme.

tomography (CT) is the modality of choice for demonstrating the exact extent of the injury[7].

Unstable injuries are likely to include at least one of the following features[8]:

- greater than 2.5 cm diastasis of the symphysis pubis;
- double, vertical or straddle fractures of the anterior pelvic arch;
- superior displacement of a fragment of any type or disruption of the pelvic ring, including double vertical fractures and/or dislocations (Malgaigne injury);
- disruption of the pelvic ring associated with a vertical fracture of the transverse process of the lowest lumbar vertebrae (this feature indicates that the integrity of the iliolumbar ligament is lost due to avulsion fracture as this ligament is a major stabilising factor of the sacroiliac joint).

Fractures of the acetabulum

These may be caused by a force through the long axis of the femur or the greater trochanter due to falling from a height[9], but more commonly

Ten

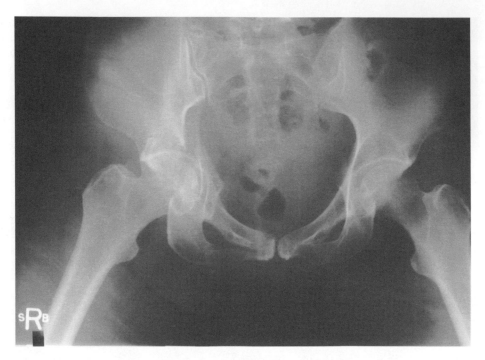

Figure 10.10   Fracture of the acetabulum and inferior pubic ramus.

as a result of a 'dashboard' injury. A dislocation or subluxation of the femoral head is associated with up to 75% of acetabular fractures. One method of classification (the Letournet–Judet classification) considers the acetabulum to be formed from two columns:

- anterior acetabular column – extending from the iliac wing to the symphysis pubis;
- posterior acetabular column – extending from the iliac wing to the ischial tuberosity.

The two columns are bridged by the acetabular roof. The medial side of the posterior column and the inner aspect of the acetabular region form the quadilateral plate.

Letournet–Judet classify acetabular fractures into four basic types, which may occur in combination[10]:

Type 1: Superior, anterior and posterior acetabular rim fractures.

Self-test answer

There is a fracture of the inferior pubic ramus and mis-alignment of the superior ramus indicative of a fracture of the region. The resting position of the latter fracture suggests acetabular involvement, best revealed by CT or further plain film projections.

Posterior most common, often associated with posterior dislocation of femoral head. CT may be required for diagnosis.

Type 2: Posterior column fractures, extending from above the acetabulum, through the posterior aspect, and often including fracture of the inferior pubic ramus.

Type 3: Anterior column fractures, starting from the anterior inferior iliac spine, through the anterosuperior acetabulum, to the obturator foramen. Often associated with pubic bone and anterior acetabular margin fractures.

Type 4: Transverse acetabular fracture crossing the acetabular fossa and involving both columns. An additional fracture line may extend caudally from the acetabular fossa, forming a 'T'-shaped fracture. Co-existing disruptions and fractures of the sacroiliac joints and pubic symphysis must be excluded.

Childhood considerations

Perthes' disease

This disease is covered in depth in Chapter 8 (p. 194). However, its uncertain aetiology of an idiopathic nature that results in presentation in the accident and emergency department indicates a need to mention the pathology here.

Slipped upper femoral epiphysis

This is one of the most significant hip disorders of adolescence and is a progressive disorder that requires early diagnosis and intervention. It is covered in Chapter 8.

Ten

References

1 Muir, L., Boot, D., Gorman, D.F., *et al.* (1996) The epidemiology of pelvic fractures in the Mersey region. *Injury* **27**(3), 199–204.
2 Gansslen, A., Pohlemann, T., Paul, C., *et al.* (1996) Epidemiology of pelvic ring injuries. *Injury* **27**(Suppl 1), S-A 13–20.
3 Hunter, J.C., Brandser, E.A. and Tran, K.A. (1997) Pelvic and acetabular trauma. *Radiologic Clinics of North America* **35**(3), 559–90.
4 De Paulis, F., Cacchio, A., Michelini, O., *et al.* (1998) Sports injuries of the pelvis and hip: diagnostic imaging. *European Journal of Radiology* **27**(Suppl 1), S49–59.
5 Whitbeck, M.G. Jr, Zwally, H.J. 2nd and Burgess, A.R. (1997) Immunosacral dissociation: mechanism of injury as a predictor of

resuscitation requirements, morbidity and mortality. *Journal of Orthopaedic Trauma* **11**(2), 82–8.

6   MacLeod, M. and Powell, J.N. (1997) Evaluation of pelvic fractures. Clinical and radiologic. *Orthopedic Clinics of North America* **28**(3), 299–319.

7   Berg, E.E., Chebuhar, C. and Bell, R.M. (1996) Pelvic trauma imaging: a blinded comparison of computed tomography and roentgenograms. *Journal of Trauma* **41**(6), 994–8.

8   Mostafavi, H.R. and Tornetta, P. 3rd. (1996) Radiologic evaluation of the pelvis. *Clinical Orthopaedics and Related Research* **Ang**(329), 6–14.

9   Pitt, M.J., Ruth, J.T. and Benjamin, J.B. (1992) Trauma to the pelvic ring and acetabulum. *Seminars in Roentgenology* **27**(4), 299–318.

10 Heller M. and Fink A. (2000) *Radiology of Trauma*, Springer-Verlag, Berlin.

Further reading

Burnett, S., Taylor, A. and Watson, M. (2000) *A–Z of Orthopaedic Radiology*. WB Saunders, London.

Manaster, B.J. (1997) *Handbooks in Radiology: Skeletal Radiology*. Mosby, London.

11 Chest Trauma

Renata Eyres and Nigel Thomas

Introduction – viewing a chest radiograph

As with all other areas of the skeleton it is important to develop a systematic approach to viewing radiographs of the chest and thoracic cavity, and to have sound knowledge of the anatomy. The anatomy and radiological appearances of the *normal* chest are extremely complex; one can only confidently diagnose an abnormality when one is completely comfortable with normal appearances. As a guide to developing a systematic approach, a checklist is provided to ensure the key areas are covered when viewing chest radiographs. This list should be read in conjunction with Figure 11.1.

- As with all radiographs, check: name, position and radiographic quality.
- Check soft-tissue areas including chest wall, breast, shoulder girdle and neck.
- Check the diaphragm region for evidence of free gas, organ size and position, calcifications, etc.
- Check the bony areas including spine and rib cage for fractures, lytic lesions, disc space narrowing, etc.
- Check the mediastinum:
  - size (particularly width) and shape;
  - position of trachea;
  - related margins – aortic arch, right atrium, left ventricle, main pulmonary artery, left subclavian artery;
  - lines and stripes, paratracheal, paraspinal, paraoesophageal, paraortic (see reference 1 for further information);
  - retrosternal space.
- Check the hilum including size, outline and density.
- Check the lungs and pleura including size, vascular markings, right to left, upper to lower, lung parenchyma, pleural surfaces (fissures, hemidiaphragm).

Figure 11.1 The normal male chest radiograph and where to view for clues to thoracic trauma.

1 = Fracture of ribs 1–3 are associated with a high incidence of mediastinal injury.

2 = Look for loss of lung markings/pleural edge for pneumothorax.

3 = Fractured ribs most commonly noted at curve apices.

4 = Widening of superior mediastinum indicates vessel rupture – take care when supine.

5 = Fluid such as blood will settle in the costophrenic angles, when erect.

6 = Elevation of the pericardium indicates pneumomediastinum.

7 = What shape is the heart shadow? Globular could indicate tamponade.

8 = Fracture of the clavicle may cause pneumothorax – assess sternoclavicular joint in more forceful injuries as there is an association with 1.

9 = Scapular fractures are rare but have strong association with 1 or 2 if evident.

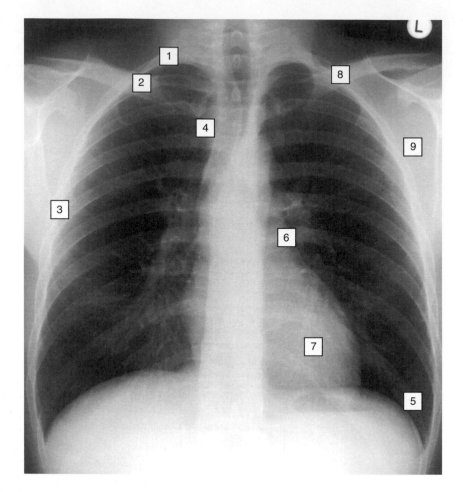

The viewer should also be aware and take account of:

- body size and shape generally;
- male or female;
- age of patient;
- possible foreign bodies or leads, lines, tubes, etc. present.

The order in which the 'search' takes place is not important, it is, however, vital that all the major structures/regions visible on the radiograph are reviewed, and that any suspected abnormality is described in detail. The types of abnormality that may be detected include:

- changes in the normal appearance of a structure;
- an area of increased density;
- an area of translucency.

Both lungs should be equally transradiant across the corresponding zones and soft tissues areas and the bony detail of structures require careful consideration.

When reviewing the diaphragm each of the following should be considered:

- The costophrenic and cardiophrenic angles:
  - ○ lateral and posterior costophrenic angles should be sharp and acute;
  - ○ cardiophrenic angles vary due to the presence of fat pads.
- Height of diaphragm:
  - ○ The right hemidiaphragm margin normally lies between the anterior ends of the fifth and seventh ribs
  - ○ In 95% of normal subjects the right hemidiaphragm is up to 3 cm higher than the left.
- Lungs and diaphragm margins should be clearly defined.
- The contour of the hemidiaphragm is generally smooth and arcuate with the highest point lying medial to the mid-lung line. The highest point on the left is usually more to the lateral aspect due to the heart.

Technical considerations

The way in which a chest radiograph has been obtained is critical for its interpretation. Particularly important is the radiographic projection. In an antero-posterior (AP) projection the heart, which lies anteriorly in the chest, is more magnified than on a postero-anterior radiograph. If the tube–film distance is also reduced on an AP projection, assessment of the heart size becomes even more difficult.

Reduced inspiration may be a sign of underlying pathology or just a lack of effort or understanding by the patient. Normally the mid-point of the right hemidiaphragm lies between the anterior ends of the fifth to the seventh ribs. Under-inflation also reduces the difference in size between the upper and lower zone vessels. Normally if the patient is examined in the erect position the lower zone vessels are larger than those in the upper zone due to gravity.

If the patient is rotated around the long axis of the body, the mediastinal structures become distorted and the radio-opacity of the right and left hemithoraces is unequal. Rotation on the horizontal coronal axis gives a more lordotic or kyphotic projection than normal which, again, may distort the mediastinal structures.

Silhouette sign

The term 'silhouette sign' is used to indicate a loss in the silhouette (the clear sharp margins; Figure 11.2) of the borders between air in the lungs

Eleven

The lung fields may likewise demonstrate pneumothorax, haemothorax or consolidation suggestive of lung contusion. Radiographic abnormalities of the mediastinum, particularly pneumomediastinum, widening of the mediastinum and shift of the mediastinum suggest airway rupture, aortic disruption and tension pneumothorax, respectively. Finally, assessment of the cardiac silhouette (cardiomegaly or pneumopericardium) may aid in the diagnosis of blunt myocardial injury including tamponade.

Rib fractures

Rib fractures can be diagnosed clinically; however, their presence indicates a need for examining the underlying lung for contusion, laceration, and haemo- or pneumothorax. Any combination of rib fractures, which can cause a part of one or more ribs to move independently of the remaining rib cage, may cause a flail segment[3]. This can be associated with serious intrathoracic injury and can also produce difficulty in artificially ventilating the patient, as paradoxical involvement of the flail segment reduces aeration of the underlying lung; this may result in respiratory failure. Fractures of the first to third ribs often indicate severe impact, as they are relatively well protected. Associated injuries may include damage to the brachial plexus, subclavian vessels, aorta or airway. Fractures of the lower ribs (tenth, eleventh, twelfth), are associated with injury to the liver (Figure 11.4), kidneys or spleen depending upon the anatomical site of injury.

Pneumothorax

Pneumothorax is an injury to the lung, either by trauma or iatrogenic cause that may result in air leaking into the pleural space. For a summary of causes see Table 11.1. A **tension pneumothorax** is a life-threatening condition, and therefore all practitioners working in an accident and emergency setting should be aware of the associated radiographic signs (see Figure 11.5). It is caused by the accumulation of air that is under pressure, within the pleural space. This in turn causes mediastinal displacement and vascular compression. A **traumatic pneumothorax** is caused by a blunt or penetrating injury and may have associated rib fractures. Mechanisms of injury include road traffic accidents, falls and penetrating wounds such as stab wounds. Surgical procedures may also result in an iatrogenic pneumothorax or a tension pneumothorax. A high index of suspicion for the presence of a pneumothorax must be maintained in all blunt trauma victims.

Haemothorax

Damage to the major thoracic vessels is important to recognise, as up to 40% of the blood volume can be accommodated in one hemithorax[5].

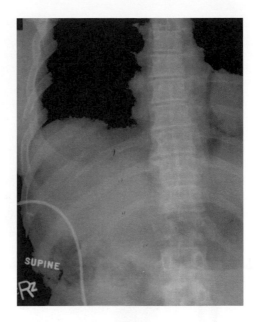

Figure 11.4 Multiple lower rib fractures.

Table 11.1   Aetiology of pneumothorax (adapted from Brant and Helms[4]).

	[Trauma]	
Iatrogenic		**Non-iatrogenic**
Thoracic/abdominal surgery		Penetrating injury
Central line placement		Stab wound
Bronchoscopy		Blunt injury
		Oesophageal rupture
		Rib fracture
	[Spontaneous]	
Primary		**Secondary**
Idiopathic		Obstructive airways disease
		Asthma
		Emphysema
		Infection
		Lung abscess
		Neoplasm
		Cystic lung disease
		Connective tissue disorders
		Marfan's syndrome

Self-test answer

Fractures of the eighth to eleventh right ribs are evident with maximal displacement of ribs 8 and 9. If clinical suspicion indicates, further examination of the liver is advised.

Eleven

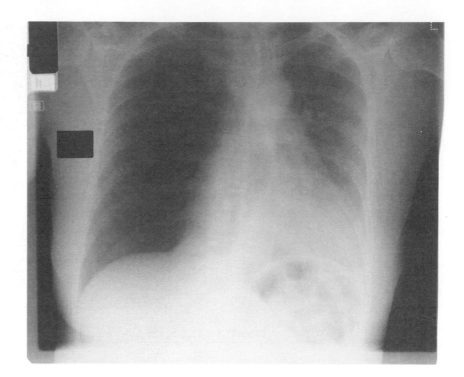

Figure 11.5 Tension pneumothorax.

Blunt injury to the lower airways is usually caused by deceleration or compression injury. These injuries typically present as a pneumothorax that does not resolve. When a haemo-pneumothorax is present, an air–fluid level can be seen on a horizontal beam lateral projection or erect PA (Figure 11.6).

Pneumomediastinum

Tracking of air or direct gas entry following a penetrating injury may generate this unusual pattern. Elevation of the pericardium is noted beneath the aorto-pulmonary window, creating a white line that is seen

Self-test answer

A large pneumothorax is seen in the right hemithorax, but also note the gross degree of mediastinal shift into the left hemithorax. The trachea is deviated significantly from its midline course. This requires immediate medical intervention.

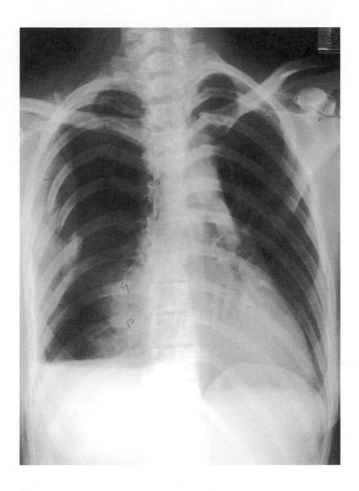

Figure 11.6 The haemopneumothorax.

on profile much like the pneumothorax pattern described above (Figure 11.7). In comparison, stabbing injuries may create a collection of blood in the pericardial sac, revealed by a globular shape of the heart shadow as the pericardium fills. Clinically the patient may display signs of cardiac arrhythmia before pressure from the filled pericardium eventually causes electro-mechanical dysfunction to cause cardiac arrest. This can only be reversed by the aspiration of the pericardium by the perceived dramatic intervention of a direct stab of the needle into the blood-filled sac.

Self-test answer

Fractures of the right fifth to eighth ribs are noted with loss of lung markings typical of a penetrating pneumothorax. A fluid level is seen in the right costophrenic region which may represent blood in the thorax.

Eleven

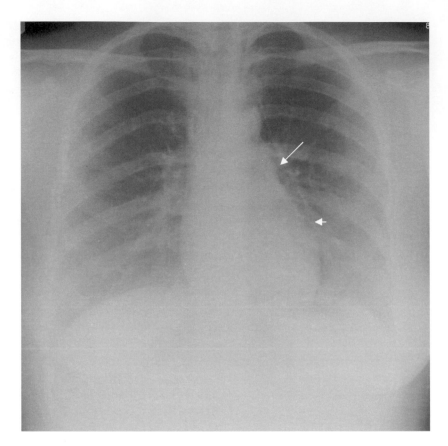

Figure 11.7 The pneumomediastinum.

Widened mediastinum

A widened mediastinum on CXR in the blunt trauma victim is usually associated with aortic injury. Several technical factors of the AP mobile film taken in the emergency setting, i.e. supine position, expiratory film and the magnification effect of a short focus-film distance, may make the mediastinum appear artefactually widened.

Aortic injury

Of patients with thoracic aortic rupture 80–90% die in the pre-hospital setting[4]. Those who survive to reach the hospital may have minimal symptoms. The chest film may give the first suggestion of injury. The rupture is usually at the isthmus just distal to the left subclavian artery, and is caused by rapid deceleration forces.

Blunt cardiac injury

Blunt trauma to the heart covers a spectrum of conditions from myocardial concussion and contusion to myocardial rupture. The right atrium and ventricle are the most frequently injured chambers because of their anterior positioning in the chest, followed by left atrium and left ventricle. Survival after one-chamber rupture is about 40%[6]. Two-chamber rupture has uniform mortality. The lower pressure in the right heart means that blood loss may be relatively slow, particularly if the pericardium is intact.

Diaphragmatic rupture

The symptoms of diaphragmatic rupture are similar to pneumothorax as the lung is compressed and hypoxaemia develops. Diagnosis is made with the help of the CXR. Loss of the diaphragmatic contour, presence of bowel or nasogastric tube in the chest or elevation of the right hemidiaphragm are all suggestive of rupture. Diaphragmatic rupture is more common on the left than the right side.

References

1   Grainger, R.G. and Allison, D.J. (eds.) (1992) *Diagnostic Radiology, An Anglo-American Textbook of Imaging, Volume 1*, 2nd edn. Churchill Livingstone, New York.
2   Heller, M. and Fink, A. (2000) *Radiology of Trauma*, Springer-Verlag, Berlin.
3   Freundlich, I.M. and Bragg, D.G. (1997) *A Radiologic Approach to Diseases of the Chest*, 2nd edn. Williams & Wilkins, Baltimore, p. 59.
4   Brant, W.E. and Helms, C.A. (1999) *Fundamentals of Diagnostic Radiology*, 2nd edn. Lippincott Williams & Wilkins, Philadelphia.
5   Devitt, J.H. (1993) Blunt thoracic trauma: anaesthesia assessment and management. *Canadian Journal of Anaesthesia* **40**(52), 29–30.
6   Perchinsky, M.J., Long, W.B. and Hill, J.G. (1993) Blunt cardiac rupture. *Archives of Surgery* **130**, 852–7.

Eleven

12 The Skull and Face

Jonathan McConnell

Introduction

There has been a gradual transition in the perception of the value of skull and facial series in the trauma situation. Difficulties in full identification of fracture components coupled with the often unco-operative condition patients present in have raised questions about the efficacy of plain film radiography. The worth of plain films becomes more questionable when head injury assessment and referral criteria are compared with other imaging modalities. Computed tomography and magnetic resonance imaging enable visualisation of soft tissue damage in the brain and provide three-dimensional information about the relationship of fracture components which is impossible with plain film imaging. However, even though the National Institute for Clinical Excellence[1,2] now recommends the use of CT for almost all head injury imaging, skull and facial examinations for fractures may still be taken in the Accident and Emergency setting. It is therefore worth considering the patterns of presentation that can be identified while recognising the limitations of this form of imaging.

It is also worth considering the skull and facial skeleton as being akin to the crumple zones of a car. If one considers the general construction of the facial skeleton, the position and shape of the strong, thick bony buttresses and the thinner plate-like structures around the orbital regions are designed to absorb forces and direct energy away from delicate structures such as the brain. Despite difficulties in generating testing procedures to demonstrate peak force and pressure fracture tolerances of individual facial bones[3], if the 'vehicle crumple' analogy is applied, how the skull functions to protect its delicate contents is readily understood.

The skull

Basic radiographs

Three main projections are drawn upon for plain film examination of the skull although variations exist[4] based on injury site, and whether all projections are used for every examination[5]. The projections are:

- **lateral** – obtained with a horizontal beam;
- **postero-anterior** (PA) or **antero-posterior** (AP) – according to patient presentation; and
- **Towne's** – shows the occipital bone but note the frontal and occipital bones are superimposed so a fracture of the frontal bone may also be seen on this projection.

Normal variants

Sutures

Position and appearance of the lambdoid, coronal and sagittal sutures should be recognised. The metopic suture, a lucent line seen on the frontal bone (created during the embryonic development of the skull) in children, may persist into adult life. Check out examples of normal variants in an atlas, e.g. by Keats *et al.* (see Further reading), if unsure. The fontanellae in the very young may also be misconstrued as manifestations of injury.

Vascular marking or fracture?

Be aware of the sites of common vessel markings. Vascular markings appear grey as only the inner surface is thinned (because vessels run only on the inner surface of the vault). Vascular markings show evidence of branching that reduce in size peripherally. Characteristically, vessel channel margins are sclerotic.

Fractures, by comparison, frequently appear black as both the inner and the outer tables of the skull are disrupted. If the fracture branches, they do not taper uniformly nor are the edges of the fracture sclerotic. However, occasions do arise when the fracture line tracks along a vascular groove such as the path of the middle meningeal artery. Where this is the case the superimposed fracture tends to darken the vascular track on the resultant radiograph – take great care to identify these injuries correctly.

Normal sphenoid sinus

In young children this sinus is not pneumatised (air filled). In adults its appearance may vary.

Twelve

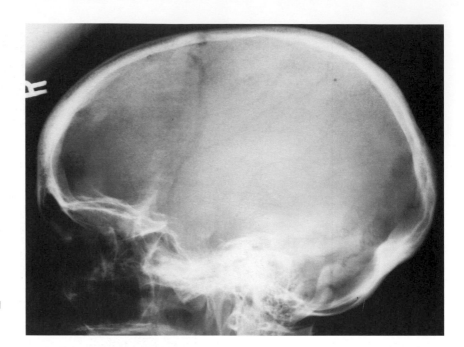

Figure 12.1 Widened coronal suture following direct blow to the head.

Abnormal plain films

It is important to check all films not only for trauma but also for pathology. A systematic approach is advised:

- intracranial calcification;
- pituitary fossa;
- bones of the vault;
- base of skull; and
- (with a bright light) the soft tissue outline.

Thus areas of lysis, sclerosis or fracture may be identified. When the history is available, closely scrutinise parts of the film corresponding to the sites of injury.

Important abnormalities

Trauma (Figure 12.1)
- Linear fractures (Figure 12.2).
- Depressed fractures appear dense due to overlying fragments (Figure 12.3).

Self-test answer

There is an apparent widening of the coronal suture that seems to extend down towards the temporal region. This appearance is consistent with a blow to the top of the head as indicated in the history.

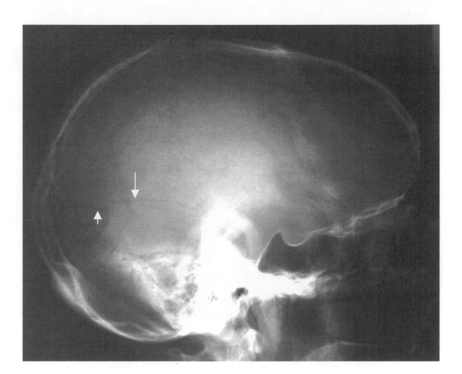

Figure 12.2 A linear fracture of the parietal region.

- Fluid level in the sphenoid sinus, if seen on the horizontal beam lateral, would indicate a basal skull fracture. This may be the only abnormality seen radiographically. A fracture that communicates with the sphenoid sinus should be considered as open and as such attract concern for future infections. Clinical clues that support this diagnosis include flow of cerebrospinal fluid (CSF) from the nose or ears or blood plus CSF from the same orifices.
- Intracranial air is seen as a lucency in the basal cisterns, the cerebral sulci or the lateral ventricles. This rare phenomenon occurs as air from a sinus fracture or penetrating wound enters the cranium (Figure 12.4).
- Lateral displacement of a calcified pineal should be no more than 3 mm to one side of the midline as seen on the AP or Towne's projection. Displacement would indicate the presence of a large

Self-test answer

A linear lucency is seen extending above and posterior to the soft tissue shadow of the ear pinna, reaching the lambdoid suture posteriorly. The appearance is indicative of a linear fracture of the parietal bone.

Twelve

(a)   (b)

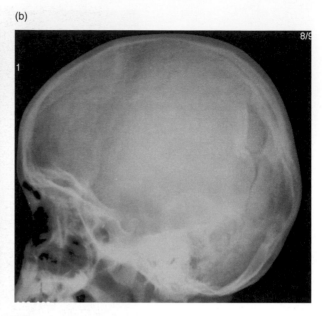

Figure 12.3   (a, b) Depressed fracture of the left parietal region.

intracranial haematoma on the opposite side of the head relative to the direction of pineal shift. Rotated films can falsely generate this appearance.

Head injuries in children may not necessarily reveal bony evidence of trauma other than as depressed fracture or penetrating injury. As many fractures may remain undetected and associated injury can be present, the use of CT is recommended to fully elucidate the extent of trauma[2].

Non-trauma

Intracranial calcification is often of no significance to the patient. Calcifications can be identified from their site; however, CT is required to diagnose correctly. Calcification is not seen in metastatic disease but may be noted in primary tumours.

Self-test answer

A lucency with apparent sclerosis around the edges is seen to lie in the left parietal region. The tangential appearance on the frontal image indicates this is a depressed fracture of the left parietal area. (Note the lack of air in the sphenoid sinus of this young patient.)

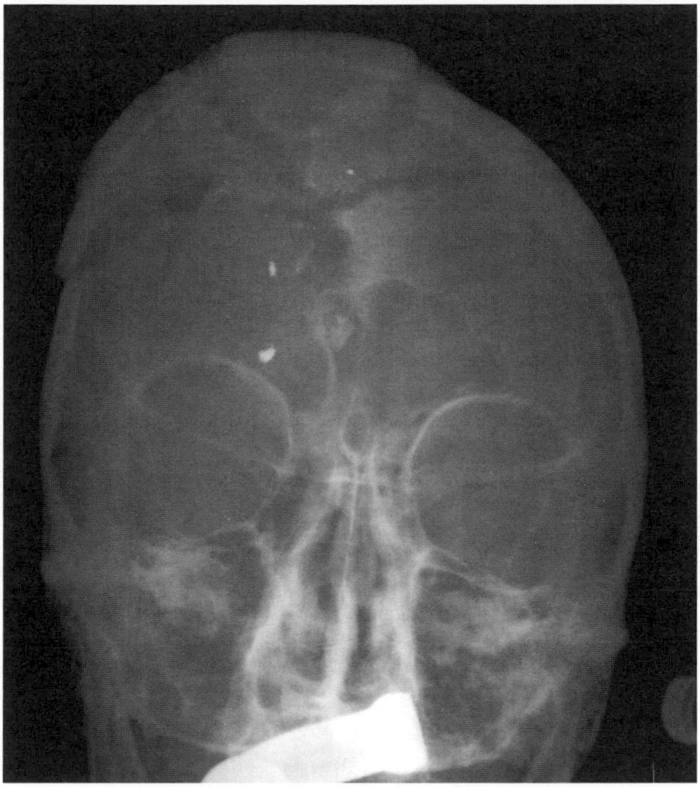

Figure 12.4 A self-inflicted gunshot wound to the head.

The facial bones

Basic radiographs

Historically, many hospitals used three projections of the facial skeleton. These included:

- **OM** – occipito-mental;
- **OM10** – occipito-mental with 10 degrees caudal angulation. Isocentric skull units may use the misleading terminology of OM30;
- Lateral.

Self-test answer

Multiple fractures are noted in the vault of the cranium with high density, possibly metallic, fragments superior to the right orbit. A metal airway is also noted to be in situ. Appearances are consistent with a self-inflicted wound to the head as suggested by the history.

Twelve

The OM-type views provide the majority of the information required to make a diagnosis of facial injury, but the lateral projection is necessary to rule out the presence of fluid levels. Although considered a useful indicator of injury, the lateral projection, it is now argued, adds little to the examination[6]. As CT is seen as the gold standard in imaging this region, arguments have been put forward for only performing a single OM projection[7,8] with full injury evaluation through use of the three-dimensional imaging modality.

For the mandible an OPT (orthopantomogram) is desirable though not always available. In these cases a PA and two oblique mandible views are options.

Theoretically, as little medical intervention is likely to take place, the nasal bones should not be radiographed unless there is airway compromise[9]. However, when requested by the appropriate clinician (ENT surgeon) a PA/OM and lateral projections may be taken.

Systematic inspection of OM projections

Systems have been devised over the years to generally guide facial injury detection on radiographs[10]. The famous **Le Fort classification**, which allows the seriousness of an injury to be described, is based on the displacement of maxillary fractures. However, with the advent of such informative techniques as reconstructive CT, this descriptive method has reduced in its authority as not all patterns are represented in the imaging.

McGrigor and Dolan's three lines

These lines tend to take the form of a 'lazy W' (see Figure 12.5).

- Line 1 – links the right and left supra-orbital margins across the frontal sinus.
- Line 2 – joins both fronto-zygomatic processes passing through the infra-orbital margins and ethmoidal sinus bases.
- Line 3 – both tempero-zygomatic processes are linked via the maxilla and nasal septal base.

When viewing the images look for the following.

- Line 1 – fractures, widening of fronto-zygomatic sutures. Remember, however, this may vary normally. Fluid levels in the frontal sinus are indicative of haemorrhage.
- Line 2 – fracture of the zygomatic arch or through the inferior rim of the orbit. A soft tissue shadow in the superior aspect of the maxillary antrum is indicative of facial swelling.
- Line 3 – fracture of the zygoma and lateral aspect of the maxillary antrum. Evidence of a fluid level in the maxillary antrum following trauma is indicative of haemorrhage.

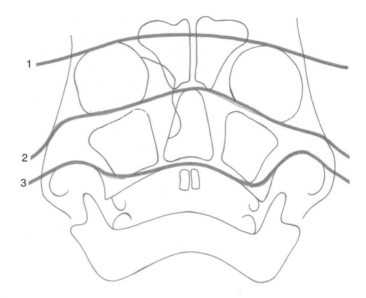

Figure 12.5 McGrigor and Dolan's lines of facial assessment. Note how the lines represent a lazy or flattened W shape that interconnects the areas of interest when reviewing the facial projections.

Le Fort's classification of facial injuries (maxillary fractures)

Although, as stated before, this classification is falling out of favour due to our understanding (through CT imaging) of what is missed on plain films, it is worth knowing what the Le Fort system describes in terms of facial injuries (Figure 12.6).

- Le Fort I – the tooth bearing part of the maxilla is separated from the remaining maxilla by a fracture through the medial and lateral walls of the maxillary sinus and nasal septum.
- Le Fort II – the separated fragment (Figure 12.7) is pyramidal with fracture lines running inferiorly and laterally through the medial and inferior walls of the orbit and then through the lateral walls of the maxillary sinuses. There is a nasal septum fracture at a variable level.
- Le Fort III – the fracture line (Figure 12.8) runs through the nasal bones in a postero-lateral direction through the medial and lateral orbital walls to exit through the zygomatic arches. The nasal septum is fractured superiorly.

A description of the main facial fractures

Tripod fracture

This injury comprises widening of the fronto-zygomatic suture, fracture of the zygomatic arch, fracture through the body of the zygoma (these features may be displayed as a fracture of the inferior orbital margin and

Twelve

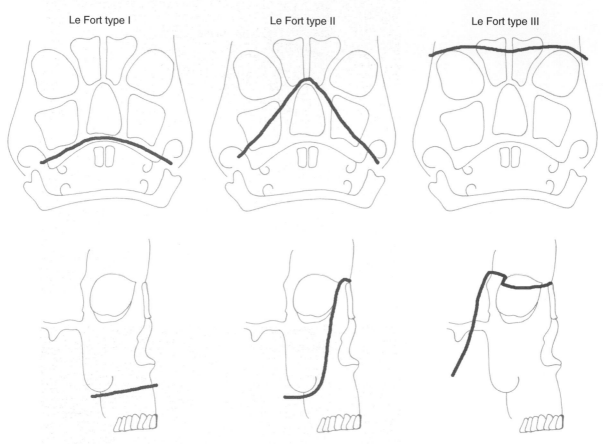

Le Fort type I   Le Fort type II   Le Fort type III

Figure 12.6   The Le Fort fracture patterns. As injury severity increases it becomes apparent that larger portions of the facial skeleton become detached from the skull.

of the lateral wall of the maxillary antrum). See Figure 12.9 – note that an isolated fracture of the zygomatic arch is common. Isolated fractures through the fronto-zygomatic suture or through the body of the zygoma rarely occur in the absence of other injuries. See Figures 12.10 and 12.11.

Blow-out fracture

This injury follows a direct compressive force to the eyeball causing fracture at the weakest point of the orbital walls due to pressure from the surrounding fat pads and rectus muscles. The standard OM-type projections[11,12] suffice to reveal the injury (as displayed in Figure 12.12) although CT will give more information following three-dimensional reconstruction.

The orbital contents (fat and inferior rectus muscle in the main) herniate down through the orbital floor[13] to create a radio-opaque 'tear-drop'

(a)

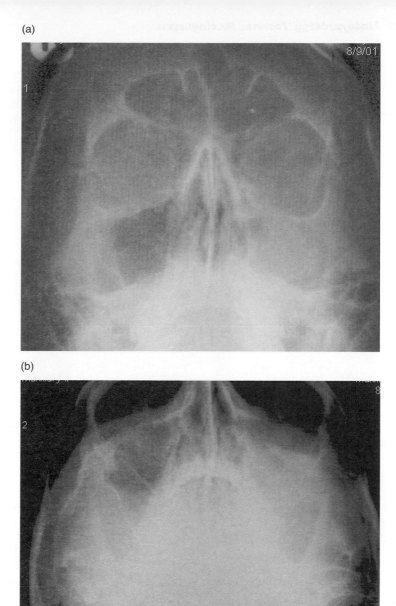

8/9/01

1

(b)

Maxillary II

Maxill

2

8

Figure 12.7 Le Fort type II
injury of the facial bones.

Self-test answer

There is a loss of radiolucency in the left maxillary sinus and
apparent widening of the fronto-zygomatic suture on the sub-
optimal OM projection. The orbital floor projection reveals a significant step on the medial side of the maxillary roof. The lateral
projection further supports the presence of fluid in the left maxillary sinus. On the right side there is an apparent loss of continuity of the lateral wall of the right maxillary sinus. All appearances
suggest fractures of the mid-facial region commensurate with a
Le Fort type II injury.

Twelve

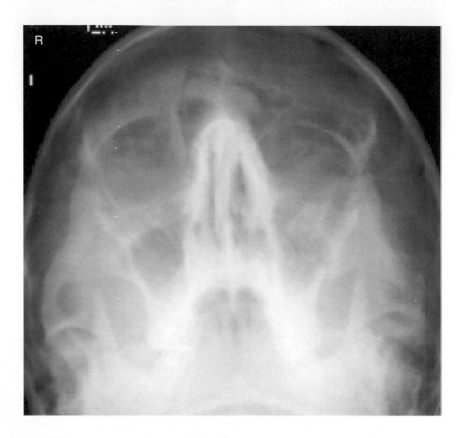

Figure 12.8   Le Fort type III injury.

appearance in the maxillary antrum as seen on the OM view. It is also possible for herniation to occur medially through the ethmoidal sinus wall.

Occasionally the teardrop cannot be seen and an ethmoidal or maxillary fracture can only be detected by the fact that air from the sinus has leaked through to enter the orbital space. The air in this instance will rise to the top of the orbit to give orbital emphysema or the 'black

Self-test answer

Both orbital margins appear deformed, the left side more markedly than the right. There are obvious steps in the left orbital floor and lateral maxillary margin, the fronto-zygomatic suture is disrupted and the zygomatic arch is fractured. Fracture lines can be discerned through the frontal sinus with an apparent fracture in the medial wall of the right orbit. These appearances are highly suggestive of a type III Le Fort injury but will require confirmation with a CT scan.

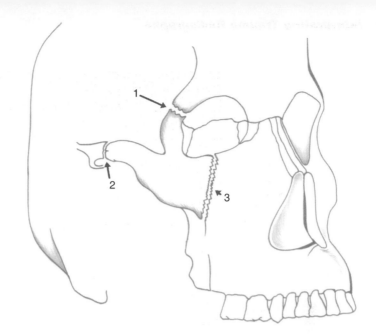

Figure 12.9 The tripod fracture. The different fracture lines are displayed representing zygomatic arch fracture (1 and 2) and inferior orbital rim injury extending through anterior and lateral walls of the maxillary antrum to the zygoma. The tripod fracture is seen with injuries at all 3 points (1–3).

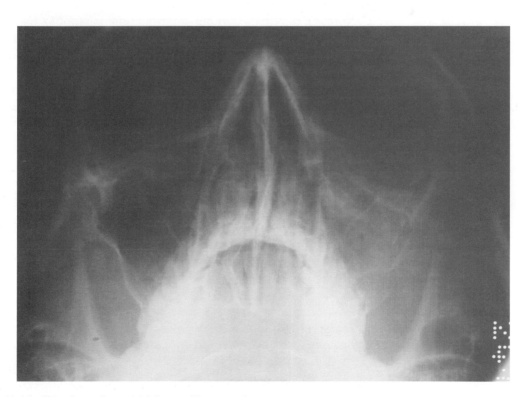

Figure 12.10 Tripod-type fracture of the maxillary complex.

Self-test answer

Gross misalignment is noted at the medial side of the left maxillary roof with extension into the lateral wall. The left fronto-zygomatic suture is disrupted consistent with a tripod-type fracture.

eyebrow' sign.[14] Note that herniation the inferior of oblique rectus muscle fat that goes undetected will result in the attachment of the muscles to the orbital margin by fibrous tissue, eventually generating a diplopia.

Maxillary fractures

These may be revealed by:

- soft tissue swelling;
- opacification of the maxillary sinus (often as a fluid level);
- soft tissue emphysema. Although rare, this is positive proof of a fracture involving the nasal cavity or sinuses. Typically seen is the

Figure 12.11   Fracture of the zygomatic arch.

Self-test answer

Gross soft tissue swelling with disruption of the normal curvature of the left zygomatic arch indicates the presence of a fracture.

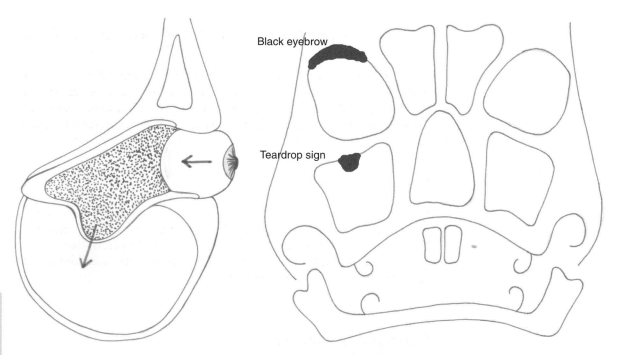

Figure 12.12   The blow-out fracture. As the orbit is forced posteriorly into the conical eye socket, the weaker bone (lamina papericia) fractures to allow mainly the fat of the lateral rectus muscle to herniate inferiorly to create the 'teardrop' sign. The 'black eyebrow' sign is generated by orbital emphysema as air leaking from a fracture of the maxillary sinus roof that forms the orbital floor rises to the top of the orbit.

Twelve

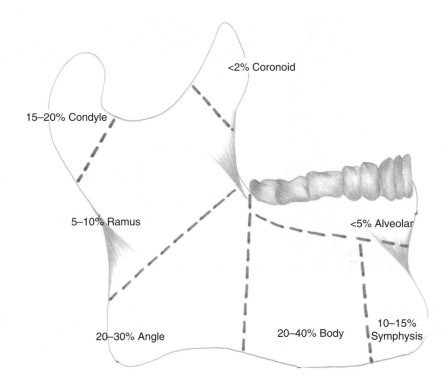

<2% Coronoid

15–20% Condyle

5–10% Ramus

<5% Alveolar

20–30% Angle

20–40% Body

10–15% Symphysis

Figure 12.13 Mandibular fractures and their prevalence.

'black eyebrow' sign or multiple radiolucent areas in the soft tissues.

The evaluation lines discussed earlier (see Figure 12.5 p. 269) are useful for scrutinising these injuries. The wearing of a maxillary denture has been linked with modification of the Le Fort I fracture pattern. In these cases a vertical fracture line is introduced which results in a communication between the base of the orbit and the maxillary sinus[15].

Mandibular fractures

If the mandible is regarded as a rigid bony ring it would be common to expect two fractures to occur at a time, as noted in other ring structures. It is wise to correlate radiological inspection with the precise site of injury as revealed clinically. Figure 12.13 demonstrates the mandibular sites and prevalence of mandibular injuries.

Concluding remarks

This chapter has given a brief overview of cranio-facial injuries to cover the major points of image patterns. Current practice appears to indicate

Twelve

that CT will be the modality of choice for full evaluation of these injuries in the future.

References

1   National Institute for Clinical Excellence (2002) Head injury in infants, children and adults: triage, assessment, investigation and early management. http://www.nice.org.uk/pdf/HI_NICE_guideline_2nd_consultation.pdf (accessed June 2003).

2   Lloyd, D.A., Carty, H., Patterson, M., *et al.* (1997) Predictive value of skull radiography for intracranial injury in children with blunt head injury. *Lancet* **349**(9055), 821–4.

3   Hampson, D. (1995) Facial injury: a review of biomechanical studies and test procedures for facial injury assessment. *Journal of Biomechanics* **28**(1), 1–7.

4   McGlinchey, I., Fleet, M.F., Eatock, F.C., *et al.* (1998) A comparison of two or threee radiographic views in the diagnosis of skull fractures. *Clinical Radiology* **53**(3), 215–17.

5   Murshid, W.R.E. (1994) Role of skull radiography in the initial evaluation of minor head injury: a retrospective study. *Acta Neurochirurgica* **129**(1–2), 11–14.

6   Raby, N. and Moore, D. (1998) Radiography of facial trauma, the lateral view is not required. *Clinical Radiology* **53**(3), 218–20.

7   Rogers, S.N., Bradley, S. and Michael, S.P. (1995) The diagnostic yield of only one occipito-mental radiograph in cases of suspected midfacial trauma – or is one enough? *British Journal of Oral and Maxillofacial Surgery* **33**(2), 90–2.

8   Sidebottom, A.J. and Lord, T.C. (1998) Single view radiographic screening of midfacial trauma. *International Journal of Oral and Maxillofacial Surgery* **27**(5), 356–7.

9   Nigam, A., Goni, A. and Benjamin, A. (1993) The value of radiographs in the management of the fractured nose. *Archives of Emergency Medicine* **10**(4), 293–7.

10 Gautam, V. and Leonard, E.M. (1994) Bony injuries in association with minor head injury: lessons for improving the diagnosis of facial fractures. *Injury* **25**(1), 47–9.

11 Iinuma, T., Hirota, Y. and Ishio, K. (1994) Orbital wall fractures. Conventional views and CT. *Rhinology* **32**(2), 81–3.

12 Rothman, M. (1997) Orbital trauma. *Seminars in Ultrasound, CT & MR* **18**(6), 437–47.

13 Erling, B.F., Iliff, N., Robertson, B., *et al.* (1999) Footprints of the globe: a practical look at the mechanism of orbital blowout fractures with a revisit to the work of Raymond Pfeiffer. *Plastic and Reconstructive Surgery* **103**(4), 1313–16.

14 Birrer, R.B., Robinson, T. and Papachristos, P. (1994) Orbital emphysema: how common, how significant? *Annals of Emergency Medicine* **24**(6), 1115–18.

Twelve

15   Cooter, R.D., Dunaway, D.J. and David, D.J. (1996) The influence of maxillary dentures on mid-facial fracture patterns. *British Journal of Plastic Surgery* **49**(6), 379–82.

Further reading

Keats, T.E. and Anderson, M.W. (2001) *An Atlas of Normal Variants that May Simulate Disease*, 7th edn. Mosby, London.

Twelve

Appendix One

Measuring performance

Most programmes of postgraduate study require the student to be able to prove they have a reporting accuracy of 90–95% agreement with the radiologist[1]. This has been achieved by using a variety of assessment methods that may be measured by receiver operator characteristics, but more usually by the evaluation of viewer scores in terms of sensitivity, specificity and accuracy. These values are calculated as shown below.

$$\textbf{Sensitivity} = \text{the ability to say abnormality is present}$$

$$= \frac{\text{True positive images}}{\text{True positive} + \text{false negative (FN)}} \times 100\%$$

$$= \frac{\text{TP}}{\text{TP} + \text{FN}} \times 100\%$$

$$\text{or} \qquad = \frac{\text{TP}}{\text{All positive images}} \times 100\%$$

where:

TP – those images perceived positive by the viewer;
TP + FN – all the actually positive images in a sample/test.

$$\textbf{Specificity} = \text{the ability to say the appearances are normal} \\ \text{(no abnormality present)}$$

$$= \frac{\text{True negative images}}{\text{True negative} + \text{false positive}} \times 100\%$$

$$= \frac{\text{TN}}{\text{TN} + \text{FP}} \times 100\%$$

$$\text{or} \qquad = \frac{\text{TP}}{\text{All positive images}} \times 100\%$$

where:

TN – those images perceived negative by the viewer;
TN + FP – all the actually negative images in a sample/test.

Accuracy

Accuracy is thus a measure of the overall ability of the viewer to say whether he or she is happy an image is positive or negative for features that would require flagging and may require intervention/treatment. It is calculated thus:

$$\text{Accuracy} = \frac{\text{Sensitivity} + \text{specificity}}{\text{Total number of images}} \times 100\%$$

$$= \frac{\text{TP} + \text{TN}}{(\text{TP} + \text{FN}) + (\text{TN} + \text{FP})} \times 100\%$$

where:

TP – total positive films seen by viewer;
TN – total negative films seen by viewer;
FP – negative films indicated as positive by viewer;
FN – positive films indicated as negative by viewer.

Reference

1 Prime, N.J., Paterson. A.M. and Henderson, P.I. (1999) The development of a curriculum – a case study of six centres providing courses in radiographic reporting. *Radiography London* 5(2), 63–70.

Appendix Two

Accessory ossicles

These are small, nodular structures usually only a few millimetres in size, that are found in various locations in the skeleton, but predominately in abundance in the foot and ankle. They are usually found alongside articular joints, embedded in tendons, and are visualised on the radiograph as they are partially ossified (they are also known as accessory centres of ossification). There is a broad variation in size and shape.

Commonly encountered ossicles of the foot:

- os trigonum: approx 50% of people have this ossicle, located posterior to the lateral tubercle of the posterior process of the talus;
- os tibiale externum: adjacent to navicular;
- os peroneum: adjacent to cuboid bone;
- ossicles of the second and fifth metatarso-phalangeal joint.

Secondary ossicles are rounded and corticated, not to be confused with a fracture which would have a lack of cortical bone at the joint margins.

Some fractures may be mistaken for accessory ossicles, such as an avulsion fracture of the base or styloid process of the fifth metatarsal. The fracture line is usually transverse to the base of the metatarsal, where the os peroneum, when present, is usually in an oblique/longitudinal orientation in relation to the base of the metatarsal.

Secondary ossification centres/unfused apophyses can be seen also in the hand and wrist. The hook of hamate arises from a secondary ossification centre and is sometimes separate from the body of the hamate. It can be differentiated from a fracture as the opposing margins of the bone are corticated. The pisiform is another bone that can cause difficulty, as it may have more than one ossification centre, which can appear similar to fracture fragments. Again, a well-corticated margin is evidence of normality.

Sesamoid bones

A pair of sesamoid bones are often seen at the head of the first metatarsal, usually bilaterally. The two bones are referred to as the tibial sesamoid (medial) and fibular sesamoid (lateral). These small bones may be bipartite, which could be confused with a fracture. However, the normal bipartite bones will have a sclerotic, intact surface, and as they are normally found bilaterally, a radiograph of the opposite side can assist with the diagnosis. The medial sesamoid bone is more often fractured than the lateral.

Unfused apophyses

An unfused apophysis can be mistaken for a fracture in children, so knowledge of the location and exact timing of ossification centres is essential.

Appendix Three

Assessment of the injured pelvis using radiographic contour lines (Judet's lines)

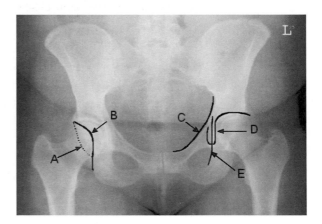

Adapted from Heller M. and Fink A. (2000) *Radiology of Trauma*, Springer-Verlag, Berlin.

Subtle fractures and disruptions of the pelvic ring and acetabulum may be difficult to visualise, especially if a trauma radiograph is not of gold-standard quality.

After assessing the radiograph for technical quality, identification and side marker, the bony landmarks and contours should be visually traced using the lines seen in the accompanying radiograph. Any disruption to the smooth contours indicates a fracture or ligamentous injury. The lines are traced as follows:

A: posterior acetabular rim

B: anterior acetabular rim

C: iliopectineal line – extends from pubic tubercle to foramen ischiadicum. Disruption of this line indicates a fracture of the anterior column of the acetabulum.

D: teardrop figure – medial limb of the teardrop corresponds to the quadrilateral surface, whereas the lateral portion represents the medial wall of the acetabulum. A continuation of this line contours the acetabular roof.

E: ilioischial line: disruption of this line represents fractures of the posterior column of the acetabulum.

Index

Index